普通高等教育"十一五"国家级规划教材

全国高等医药院校药学类专业第二轮实验双语教材

药物化学实验与指导

（第2版）

主　　编　尤启冬

副 主 编　李志裕

编　　者　（以姓氏笔画为序）

尤启冬　卞金磊　朱启华　江　程

李志裕　徐云根　徐晓莉　郭小可

U0206152

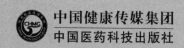
中国健康传媒集团

中国医药科技出版社

内容提要

　　本教材为"全国高等医药院校药学类专业第二轮实验双语教材"之一，是中英文对照实验类教材。上版教材被评为教育部"普通高等教育'十一五'国家级规划教材"。与上一版教材相比，本版教材保留了原有的 9 个实验，新增了 7 个实验，由原有的 12 个实验增加为 16 个实验。本书为书网融合教材，即纸质教材有机融合电子教材、数学配套资源、数字化教学服务（在线教学、在线作业、在线考试），使教学资源更加多样化、立体化。本教材适合本科药学类、制药类等专业使用。

图书在版编目（CIP）数据

药物化学实验与指导：中英／尤启冬主编. —2 版. —北京：中国医药科技出版社，2021.5
全国高等医药院校药学类专业第二轮实验双语教材
ISBN 978 - 7 - 5214 - 2167 - 5

Ⅰ. ①药⋯　Ⅱ. ①尤⋯　Ⅲ. ①药物化学 - 化学实验 - 双语教学 - 医学院校 - 教学参考资料
Ⅳ. ①R914 - 33

中国版本图书馆 CIP 数据核字（2020）第 235228 号

美术编辑　陈君杞
版式设计　南博文化

出版　**中国健康传媒集团** | 中国医药科技出版社
地址　北京市海淀区文慧园北路甲 22 号
邮编　100082
电话　发行：010 - 62227427　邮购：010 - 62236938
网址　www.cmstp.com
规格　889 × 1194mm $\frac{1}{16}$
印张　10 $\frac{1}{4}$
字数　256 千字
初版　2003 年 7 月第 1 版
版次　2021 年 5 月第 2 版
印次　2024 年 7 月第 3 次印刷
印刷　三河市万龙印装有限公司
经销　全国各地新华书店
书号　ISBN 978 - 7 - 5214 - 2167 - 5
定价　**40.00 元**

获取新书信息、投稿、为图书纠错，请扫码联系我们。

　　教学是学校人才培养的中心环节，实验教学是这一环节的重要组成部分。"全国高等医药院校药学类专业第二轮实验双语教材"是中国药科大学坚持药学实践教学改革，突出提高学生动手能力、创新思维，通过承担教育部"世行贷款21世纪初高等教育教学改革项目"等多项教改课题，逐步建设完善的一套与药学各专业学科理论课程紧密结合的高水平双语实验教材。

　　本轮修订，适逢"全国高等医药院校药学类专业第五轮规划教材"及《中国药典》（2020年版）、新版《国家执业药师资格考试大纲》出版，整套教材的修订强调了与新版理论教材知识的结合，与《中国药典》（2020年版）等新颁布的法典法规结合。为更好地服务于新时期高等院校药学教育与人才培养的需要，在上一版的基础上，进一步体现了各门实验课程自身独立性、系统性和科学性，又充分考虑到各门实验课程之间的联系与衔接，主要突出了以下特点。

　　1. 适应医药行业对人才的要求，体现行业特色，契合新时期药学人才需求的变化，使修订后的教材符合《中国药典》（2020年版）等国家标准及新版《国家执业药师资格考试大纲》等行业最新要求。

　　2. 更新完善内容，打造教材精品。在上版教材基础上进一步优化、精炼和充实内容。紧密结合"全国高等医药院校药学类专业第五轮规划教材"，强调与实际需求相结合，进一步提高教材质量。

　　3. 为适应信息化教学的需要，本轮教材全部打造成为书网融合教材，即纸质教材与数字教材、配套教学资源、题库系统、数字化教学服务有机融合，为读者提供全免费增值服务。

　　4. 坚持双语体系，强调素质培养教材以实践教学为突破口，采用双语体系编写有利于加快药学教育国际接轨，提高学生的科技英语水平，进一步提升学生整体素质。

　　"全国高等医药院校药学类专业第二轮实验双语教材"历经15年4次建设，在各个时期广大编者的努力下，在广大使用教材师生的支持下日臻完善。本轮教材的出版，必将对推动新时期我国高等药学教育的发展产生积极而深远的影响。希望广大师生在教学实践中对本套教材提出宝贵意见，以便今后进一步修订完善，共同打造精品教材。

吴晓明

全国高等医药院校药学类专业第五轮规划教材常务编委会主任委员

2019年10月

Since its first edition was published in 2000, *Experiment and Guide for Medicinal Chemistry* (*Experiment and Guide*) has been used by teachers and students for 20 years. And its demand has not abated because it is dedicated to improve the teaching and learning process for the undergraduate students. In 2007, in order to implement the bilingual education demanded by the ministry of education, we revised and published the bilingual edition (the second edition) of "*Experiment and Guide for Medicinal Chemistry*" based on the first edition. This *Experiment and Guide* is listed as "the bilingual experimental textbook of pharmacy in the national higher medical colleges and universities", and is named "the National Planning Textbook for General Higher Educationin during 'the 11th Five – Year Plan'" by the Ministry of Education. This time, in order to adapt the requirements of the country and society for the cultivation of undergraduate students in innovative and entrepreneurial talents, we revised and compiled the third edition of the bilingual *Experiment and Guide* on the basis of the second edition.

Compared with the second edition of the textbook, this "*Experiment and Guide for Medicinal Chemistry*" retains the original 9 experiments, and newly adds 7 experiments, and the total experimental numbers increase from the 12 to 16. The newly adding experiments expand the types of drugs in clinical, involved some new approved drugs in the recent years and innovative drugs researched and developed by China. These new experiments could broaden the students' horizons and match the requirement of innovative entrepreneurial talent training. Some of the new experiments have been applied in our experimental training for undergraduates and some of them come from the research results of open experiments and innovative projects of college students. These new experiments have relatively strong application. In the third edition, we gave out ^1H – NMR and HSMS spectrum for each drug to train the students' ability for structure elucidation of the synthesized drugs, and the HPLC methods of drug purity determination for students to have a concept of drug quality.

When the "*Experiment and Guide for Medicinal Chemistry*" was used by the other colleges and universities, they could select the suitable experiments from it for their students' teaching and ability training, according to their own conditions, or combined with innovative entrepreneurial projects.

Experiments 1 to 9 in this third edition are the retaining parts of the second edition, and experiments 10 to 16 are newly adding parts. The experimental operations of experiment 1 to experiment 5 were also recorded in video with bilingual explanation in English and Chinese, which can be used for the reference of each school. Since the limitation of the editor's English level, there must be a lot of inaccurate expression, please it is encouraged that the readers and users could tell us and help to correct it in time.

The final desire of our editors is to make *Experiment and Guide for Medicinal Chemistry* become the reference book of experiment techniques rather than simply a teaching book of experimentation. The editors have made great effort in compiling this book, however, mistakes would not be avoided because of advance knowledge, suggestions and comments are always welcome.

Editor

August 2020

《药物化学实验与指导》一书自 2000 年编写出版以来，已有 20 年时间。这本教材在使用中受到广大师生的欢迎，在教学过程中发挥了重要作用。2007 年，为贯彻教育部有关双语教学的要求，我们在原有实验教材的基础上，修订出版了《药物化学实验与指导》的双语教材。该教材被列为"全国高等医药院校药学类实验双语教材"，被评为教育部"普通高等教育"十一五"国家级规划教材"。此次，为适应国家和社会对创新创业人才培养的需要，我们在上版实验教材的基础上，进行修订，编写了第二版《药物化学实验与指导》的双语教材。

与上一版教材相比，本教材保留了原有的 9 个实验，新增了 7 个实验，由原有的 12 个实验增加为 16 个实验。新增的实验内容拓展了实验所涉及药物的类别，特别是在新增的药物中既有近年来新上市的药物，也有我国自主研发创新药物，既开拓学生视野，满足创新创业人才能力培养的需求；同时也在实验教学过程中让学生对我国自主研发的新药有具体的认知，增强民族自豪感。新增的实验有些已在我们的教学中进行了应用，有些是来自于大学生开放实验和创新项目的研究成果，应用性比较强。此次修订，我们还在每个药物的实验中，给出该药物的 ^1H-NMR 和 HSMS 图谱，以培养学生对所合成药物结构的解析能力；给出了药物纯度测定的 HPLC 方法，让学生有一个药品质量的概念。该教材适用于药学类、制药类各专业本科生的药物化学课程实验教学，各高校还可根据自身的条件，或结合大学生创新创业项目，有选择性地用于学生的教学和能力培养。

本教材的实验一至实验九是原实验教材中的内容，实验十至实验十六是新增内容。实验一至实验五还拍制了实验录像，并配有中英文双语的解说，可供各学校教学参考。

本实验教材的编写者都是来自中国药科大学药学院药物化学系从事实验教学一线的中、青年教师。李志裕教授负责第二部分中的实验一、实验四、实验十和实验十二的编写；徐云根教授负责实验六、实验七和实验八的编写；江程教授负责实验五和实验十六的编写；郭小可副教授负责实验三和实验十三的编写；卜金磊副教授负责实验二和实验十五的编写；朱启华副教授负责实验九和实验十一的编写；徐晓莉副教授负责实验十四的编写。尤启冬教授负责第一部分和附录及全书中、英文的规范和校核工作。

本书的编写只是一个尝试，我们希望该书不仅是一本实验教学用书，也是一本实验技术参考书，若能达到此目的，也算是实现我们最终的愿望。尽管编者在编写过程中，作出了认真的努力，但由于水平有限，若有疏漏和不妥之处，敬请各位同仁及广大读者提出宝贵意见。

编　者
2020 年 8 月

第一部分　实验室基本知识

一、实验室安全

药物化学和有机化学一样是一门实践性很强的学科，因此，在进入实验室工作之前，希望参加实验者必须对实验课程的内容，要有充分的准备，而且要通晓实验室的一些基本规则，遵守实验室安全操作须知，才能避免可能发生的一些危险情况。

（一）眼睛安全防护

在实验室中，眼睛是最容易受到伤害的。飞溅出的腐蚀性化学药品和化学试剂，进入眼睛会引起灼伤和烧伤；在操作过程中，溅出的碎玻璃片或某些固体颗粒，也会使眼睛受到伤害；更有甚者，有可能发生的爆炸事故，更容易使眼睛受到损伤。因此在实验室中，最重要的是要佩戴合适的防护目镜。防护目镜一般是有机玻璃的并有护眶，可以遮挡住整个眼睛。为了安全起见，在进入实验室后要养成戴护目镜的习惯。

倘若有化学药品或酸、碱液溅入眼睛，应赶快到水龙头下，用大量的水冲洗眼睛和脸部，并赶快到最近的医院进行治疗。若有固体颗粒或碎玻璃粒进入眼睛内，请切记不要揉眼睛，立即去有关医院进行诊治。

（二）预防火灾

有机药物合成实验室中，由于经常使用挥发性的、易燃性的各种有机试剂或溶剂，最容易发生的危险就是火灾。因此在实验中应严格遵守实验室的各项规章制度，从而可以预防火灾的发生。

在实验室或实验大楼内禁止吸烟。实验室中使用明火时应考虑周围的环境，如周围有人使用易燃易爆溶剂时，应禁用明火。

一旦发生火灾，不要惊慌，须迅速切断电源、熄灭火源，并移开易燃物品就近寻找灭火的器材，扑灭着火。对容器中少量溶剂起火，可用石棉网、湿抹布或玻璃盖住容器口，扑灭着火；其他着火，采用灭火器进行扑灭，并立即报告有关部门或打 119 火警电话报警。

在实验中，万一衣服着火了，切勿奔跑，否则火借风势会越烧越烈，可就近找到灭火喷淋器或自来水龙头，用水冲淋使火熄灭。

（三）割伤、烫伤和试剂灼伤处理

1. 割伤　遇到割伤时，如无特定的要求，应用水充分清洗伤口，并取出伤口中碎玻璃或残留固体，用无菌的绷带或创可贴进行包扎、保护。大伤口应注意压紧伤口或主血管，进行止血，并立即送医院进行处理。

2. 烫伤　因火焰或因触及灼热物体所致的小范围的轻度烫伤、烧伤，可通过立即将受伤部位浸入冷水或冰水中约 5 分钟以减轻疼痛。重度的大范围的烫伤或烧伤应立即去医院进行救治。

1

3. 化学试剂灼伤 对于不同的化学试剂灼伤，处理的方法不一样。

（1）酸 立即用大量水冲洗，再用3%～5%碳酸氢钠溶液淋洗，最后水洗10～15分钟。严重者将灼伤部位拭干包扎好，送到医院治疗。

（2）碱 立即用大量水冲洗再用2%醋酸溶液、25%醋溶液，或1%硼酸溶液淋洗，以中和碱，最后再水洗10～15分钟。

（3）溴 立即用大量水冲洗，再用10%硫代硫酸钠溶液淋洗或用湿的硫代硫酸钠纱布覆盖灼伤处，至少3小时。

（4）有机物 用酒精擦洗可以除去大部分有机物。然后再用肥皂和温水洗涤即可。如果皮肤被酸等有机物灼伤。将灼伤处浸在水中至少3小时，然后请医生处置。

（四）中毒预防

有毒物质溅入口中尚未咽下者应立即吐出，用大量水冲洗口腔。如已吞下，应根据毒物性质进行解毒，并立即送医院救治。

刺激性及神经性毒物中毒，先用牛奶或鸡蛋白使之冲淡或缓和，再设法催吐，使误入口中的毒物吐出，并送医院救治。

吸入气体中毒者，将中毒者移至室外通风处，解开衣领或纽扣，使其呼吸新鲜空气，必要时实施人工呼吸。

二、化学药品、试剂的存储及使用

（一）化学药品的贮存

一般实验室中不应存储过多的化学药品和试剂，一般应实行"需要多少，领用多少"的原则。在大多数情况下，实验室所用的化学药品都贮存在带磨口塞（最好是标准磨口）的玻璃瓶内，高黏度的液体放在广口瓶中，一般性液体存放在细颈瓶内，氢氧化钠和氢氧化钾的溶液保存在带橡皮塞或塑料塞的瓶内。对于能够与玻璃发生反应的化合物（如氢氟酸），则使用塑料或金属容器，碱金属存放在煤油中，黄磷则需以水覆盖。

对光敏感的物质，包括醚在内，都有形成过氧化物的倾向，在光线的作用下更是如此，应将它们贮存在棕色玻璃瓶中。

对产生毒性或腐蚀性蒸气的物质（如溴、发烟硫酸、盐酸、氢氟酸），建议放在通风橱内专门的地方。

少量的或对潮湿气和空气敏感的物质常密封贮存于玻璃安瓿中。

某些毒品（如氰化物、砷及其化合物等）应按有关部门的规定进行贮存。

（二）化学药品使用中注意的事项

有机溶剂具有易燃和有毒两个特点。

易燃的有机溶剂（特别是低沸点易燃溶剂）在室温时有较大的蒸气压，当空气中混杂易燃有机溶剂的蒸气达到某一极限时，遇到明火即会发生燃烧爆炸。而且有机溶剂蒸气都较空气的比重大，会沿着桌面或地面飘移至较远处，或沉积在低洼处。因此，在实验室中用剩的火柴梗切勿乱丢，以免引起火灾。也不要将易燃溶剂倒入废物缸中，更不能用开口容器盛放易燃溶剂。

有机溶剂以较为隐蔽的方式产生对人的毒害，在使用中应注意最大限度地减少与有机溶剂的直接接触，不要掉以轻心。实验室中应妥善通风。在规范、小心的操作下，有机溶剂不致造成任何健康问题。操作有毒试剂和物质时，必须戴上橡皮手套或一次性塑料手套。操作后立即洗手。注意切勿让有毒物质触及五官或伤口。

三、废品的销毁

碎玻璃和其他锐角的废物不要丢入废纸篓或类似的盛器中，应该用一只专门的废物箱。

不要把任何用剩的试剂倒回到试剂瓶中，因为其一是会对试剂造成污染，影响其他人的实验；其二是由于操作疏忽导致错误引入异物，有时会发生剧烈的化学反应甚至会引起爆炸。

危险的废品，例如放出毒气或能够自燃的废品（如活性镍、磷、碱金属），决不能丢弃在废物箱或水槽中。不稳定的化学品和不溶于水或与水不混溶的溶液也禁止倒入下水道，应将它们分类集中后处理；对倒掉后能与水混溶，或能被水分解，或为腐蚀性液体时，必须用大量的水冲洗。

金属钾或钠的残渣应分批小量地加到大量的醇中予以分解（必须戴防护镜）。

四、实验记录和报告

做好实验记录和实验报告是每一个科研人员必备的基本素质。实验记录应记在专门的实验记录本上，实验记录本应有连续页码。所有观察到的现象、实验时间、原始数据、操作和后处理方法、步骤均应及时、准确、详细地记录在实验记录本上，并签上名，以保证实验记录的完整性、连续性和原始性。任何将实验情况记录在便条纸、餐巾纸、纸巾等容易遗落或损失的地方的做法都是错误的。

在实验前，对所做的实验应该充分做好预习工作。预习工作包括：反应的原理，可能发生的副反应，反应机制，实验操作的原理和方法，产物提纯的原理和方法，注意事项及实验中可能出现的危险及处置办法。应给出详细的报告。同时还要了解反应中化学试剂的化学计量学用量，对化学试剂和溶剂的理化常数等要记录在案，以便查询。

如下所示是常见的实验记录格式。

实验题目：

实验人： 实验日期： 天气： 室温：

一、实验目的

二、反应原理

三、可能发生的副反应

四、化学试剂规格及用量

五、实验操作

六、小结

第二部分 药物合成实验

实验一 诺氟沙星的合成

【实验目的】

1. 通过对诺氟沙星合成工艺的研究，使学生对新药研制过程有一个基本认识。

2. 通过对诺氟沙星合成路线的比较，使学生掌握选择实际生产工艺的几个基本原则。

3. 通过实际操作，对涉及到的各类反应特点、机制、操作要求、反应终点的控制等，进一步巩固有机化学实验的基本操作，领会理论知识。

4. 掌握各步中间体的质量控制方法。

【实验原理】

诺氟沙星（norfloxacin）的化学名为 1 - 乙基 - 6 - 氟 - 1，4 - 二氢 - 4 - 氧 - 7 - （1 - 哌嗪基）- 3 喹啉羧酸，[1 - ethyl - 6 - fluoro - 1，4 - dihydro - 4 - oxo - 7 - （1 - piperazinyl）- 3 - quindinecarboxylic acid]。化学结构式为：

诺氟沙星为微黄色针状晶体或结晶性粉末，熔点 216 ~ 220℃，易溶于酸及碱，微溶于水、丙酮和乙醇。

诺氟沙星的制备方法很多，按不同原料及路线划分可有十几种，但在我国工业生产以下述路线为主。将氟氯苯胺与乙氧基次甲基丙二酸二乙酯（EMME）高温缩合、环合，得 6 - 氟 - 7 - 氯 - 1，4 - 二氢 - 4 - 氧喹啉羧酸乙酯（1 - 3），用溴乙烷乙基化，得 1 - 乙基 - 6 - 氟 - 7 - 氯 - 1，4 - 二氢 - 4 - 氧 - 喹啉 - 3 - 羧酸乙酯（1 - 4），然后水解，再与醋酐和硼酸形成的（AcO)₃B 反应生成硼螯合物（1 - 5），（1 - 5）在 DMSO 中与哌嗪缩合，最后经 NaOH 水解得诺氟沙星。

（结构式图示）

诺氟沙星

【实验预习】

1. 对于该反应，请找出其他的乙基化试剂并简述其优缺点。

2. 该反应的副产物是什么，简述减少副产物的方法。

3. 采用何种方法可使溴乙烷得到最充分合理的应用？

4. （1-4）的合成中，减压回收 DMF 后，如果不降温，加水稀释，对反应有何影响？

【知识点】

仪器装置，投料过程，缩合反应，环合反应，水解反应，重结晶，纯度检查。

【实验步骤】

（一）7-氯-6-氟-1，4-二氢-4-氟喹啉-3-羧酸乙酯（1-3）的制备

1. 原料规格及配比 见表 1-1。

表 1-1 原料规格及配比表

原料名称	规格	用量	摩尔数	摩尔比
4-氟-3-氯苯胺（1-1）	工业品	15g	0.103	1
EMME	工业品	24g	0.111	1.07
石蜡油	CP	80ml		
甲苯	CP			
丙酮	CP			

2. 实验操作 在装有搅拌、回流冷凝器、温度计装置的三颈瓶（附注 1）中分别投入 4-氟-3-氯苯胺（1-1）、EMME，快速搅拌下加热到 120℃，于 120~130℃下反应 2 小时，放冷至室温，将回流装置改成蒸馏装置，加入石蜡油 80ml，加热到 260~270℃（附注 2），有大量乙醇生成，回收乙醇反应半小时后，冷却到 60℃下过滤，滤饼分别用甲苯、丙酮洗至滤饼呈灰白色，烘干测熔点，mp. 297~298℃，计算收率（附注 3）。

3. 附注

（1）本反应为无水反应，所有仪器应干燥，严格按无水反应操作，否则少量水分会导致 EMME 的分解。

（2）环合温度应控制在 260~270℃，为避免温度超过 270℃，可在将要到达 270℃时缓

缓加热；反应开始后，反应液变得黏稠，为避免局部过热，应快速搅拌。

（3）该环合反应是典型的 Gould-Jacobs 反应，考虑苯环上的取代基的定位效应及空间效应，3 位氯的对位远比邻位活泼，但亦不能忽略邻位的取代，条件控制不当便会按下式反应形成反环物。

为减少反环物的生成应注意以下几点：①反应温度低，有利于反环物的生成。文献报道在低温下反应可得到产物与反环物的相对含量为 1∶1 的混合物。因此反应温度应快速达到 260℃，且保持反应在 260～270℃反应。②加大溶剂用量可以降低反环物的生成。表 1-2 中一组溶剂用量与产物比例的实验数据，从经济的角度说明采用溶剂与反应物量比 3∶1 时比较合适，如表 1-2 所示。③用二苯醚或二苯砜为溶剂时，会减少反环物的生成，但价格昂贵。亦可用价廉的工业柴油代替石蜡油。

表 1-2　溶剂与反应物的用量比对反应收率的影响

溶剂与反应物的用量比	产物与反环物的比例	总收率
1	81.6∶18.4	97.2
3	85.5∶14.5	95.4
8	94.7∶5.3	96.4

4. 思考题

（1）请写出 Gould-Jacobs 反应历程，并讨论何种反应条件有利于提高产物收率。

（2）本反应为高温反应，试举出几种高温浴装置，并写出安全注意事项。

（二）1-乙基-7-氯-6-氟-1,4-二氢-4-氧喹啉-3-羧酸乙酯（1-4）的制备

1. 原料规格及配比　见表 1-3。

表 1-3　原料规格及配比表

原料名称	规格	用量	摩尔数	摩尔比
环合物（1-3）	上一步自制	25g	0.093	1
溴乙烷	CP	25g	0.229	2.46
DMF	CP	125g		
碳酸钾	CP	30.8g	0.223	2.39

2. 实验操作　在装有搅拌器、回流冷凝器、温度计、滴液漏斗的 250ml 四颈瓶中，投入环合物（1-3）、无水碳酸钾、DMF（附注 1），搅拌加热到 70℃，于 70%～80℃下，在 40～60 分钟内滴加溴乙烷（附注 2），升温至 100～110℃，保温 6～8 小时，反应完后，减压回收 70%～80% 的 DMF，降温至 50℃左右，加入 200ml 水（附注 3），析出固体（附注 4），过滤，水洗（附注 5），干燥得粗品，用乙醇重结晶（附注 6）。mp.144～145℃，计算收率。

3. 附注

（1）反应中所用 DMF 要预先进行干燥，少量水分对收率有很大影响，所用无水碳酸钾须炒过。

（2）溴乙烷沸点低，易挥发，为避免损失，可将滴液漏斗的滴管加长，插到液面以下，同时注意反应装置密闭性。

（3）反应液加水时要降温至50℃左右；而温度太高导致酯键水解，过低会使产物结块，不易处理。

（4）环合物在溶液中酮式与烯醇式有一平衡，反应后可得到少量 O-乙基化合物，该化合物随主产物一起进入以后的反应，使生成6-氟-1，4-二氢-4-氧代-7-（1-哌嗪基）喹啉（简称脱羧物），成为诺氟沙星中的主要杂质。不同的乙基化试剂，O-乙基产物生成量不一样，采用 EtBr 时较低。

O-乙基产物

脱羧物

（5）滤饼洗涤时要将颗粒碾细，同时用大量水冲洗，否则会有少量 K_2CO_3 残留。

（6）乙醇重结晶操作过程。取粗品，加入4倍量的乙醇，加热至沸，溶解，稍冷，加入活性炭，回流10分钟，趁热过滤，滤液冷却至10℃结晶析出，过滤，洗涤干燥得精品，测熔点（mp. 144～145℃）。母液中尚有部分产品，可以浓缩一半体积后，冷却，析晶，所得产品亦可用于下步投料。

4. 思考题

（1）对于该反应，请找出其他的乙基化试剂并简述其优缺点。

（2）该反应的副产物是什么？简述减少副产物的方法。

（3）采用何种方法可使溴乙烷得到最充分合理的应用？

（4）如减压回收 DMF 后，不降温，加水稀释，对反应有何影响？

（三）硼螯合物（1-5）的制备

1. 原料规格及配比　见表1-4。

表1-4　原料规格及配比表

原料名称	规格	用量	摩尔数	摩尔比
乙基物（1-4）	上一步自制	10g	0.034	1
硼酸	CP	3.3g	0.053	1.54
醋酐	CP	17g	0.167	4.9
氯化锌	CP	1g		
乙醇	CP	适量		

2. 实验操作　在装有搅拌、冷凝器、温度计、滴液漏斗的750ml四颈瓶中，加氯化锌、硼酸及少量醋酐（附注1），搅拌加至79℃，反应引发后，停止加热，自动升温至120℃，滴加剩余醋酐，加完后回流1小时，冷却，加入乙基物（1-4），回流2.5小时，冷却到室温，加水，过滤，少量冰乙醇洗至灰白色（附注2），烘干，测熔点，mp. 275℃（分解）。

3. 附注

（1）硼酸与醋酐反应生成硼酸三乙酰酯。

$$3Ac_2O + H_3BO_3 \longrightarrow (AcO)_3B$$

此反应到达79℃即其反应临界点时才开始反应，并放出大量热，温度急剧升高；如果量大有冲料的危险，故建议使用250ml以上的反应瓶，并缓缓加热。

（2）由于螯合物在乙醇中有一定溶解度，为避免产品损失，最后洗涤时，可先用冰水洗涤，温度降下来后，用冰乙醇洗。

4. 思考题

（1）搅拌快慢对该反应有何影响？

（2）加入乙基物后，反应体系中主要有哪几种物质？

（四）诺氟沙星的制备

1. 原料规格及配比　见表1-5。

表1-5　原料规格及配比表

原料名称	规格	用量	摩尔数	摩尔比
螯合物（1-5）	上一步自制	10g	0.025	1
无水哌嗪	CP	8g	0.116	4.64
二甲亚砜（DMSO）	CP	30g		
NaOH（10%）		20ml		
乙酸	CP	适量		

2. 实验操作　在装有搅拌、回流冷凝器、温度计的150ml三颈瓶中，加螯合物（1-5）（附注1）、无水哌嗪DMSO，于110℃反应3小时，冷却至90℃，加入10% NaOH，回流2小时（附注2），冷至室温，加50ml水稀释，乙酸调pH等于7.2，过滤，水洗（附注3），得粗品。在100ml烧杯中加入粗品、100ml水，用HAc调至pH 4~5，析出产品，过滤，水洗，干燥，得诺氟沙星，测熔点，mp. 216~220℃。

3. 附注

（1）硼螯合物可以利用4位羰基氧的p电子向硼原子轨道转移的特性，增强诱导效应、激活7-Cl、钝化6-F，从而选择性地提高哌嗪化收率，能彻底地防止氯哌酸的产生。

（2）由于诺氟沙星溶于碱，如反应液在加入NaOH回流后澄清，表示反应已进行完全。

（3）过滤粗品时，要将滤饼中的醋酸盐洗净，防止将其带入精制过程，影响产品的质量。

4. 思考题　从该反应的特点出发，选择几种可以替代DMSO的溶剂或溶剂系统。

【诺氟沙星的结构表征】

熔点：218~224℃。

^1H-NMR：结构正确（附图1-1）。

HRMS（ESI$^+$）：320.1055（M+H$^+$）（附图1-2）。

HPLC纯度：99.9%

HPLC测试的色谱条件：

色谱柱：十八烷基硅烷键合硅胶（4.6mm×250mm，5μm）。

流速：1.0ml/min。

进样量：10μl。

检测波长：278nm。

流动相：以 0.025mol/L 磷酸溶液（用三乙胺调节 pH 至 3.0±0.1）－乙腈（87∶13）为流动相 A，乙腈为流动相 B；按表 1－6 进行线性梯度洗脱。使用前需超声脱气。

表 1－6　洗脱表

时间/min	流动相 A/%	流动相 B/%
0	100	0
10	100	0
20	50	50
30	50	50
32	100	0
42	100	0

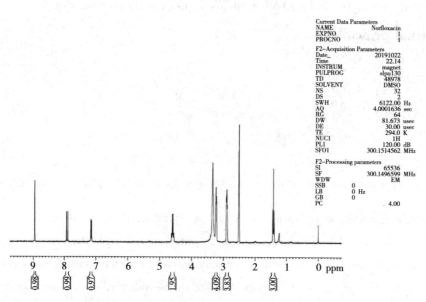

附图 1－1　诺氟沙星的 ^{1}H－NMR 谱图（DMSO－d$_6$）

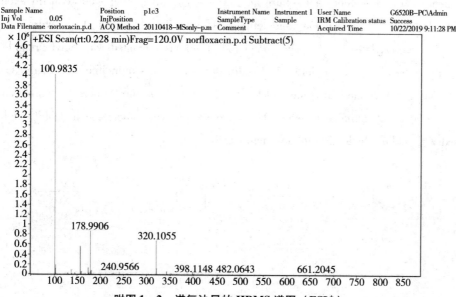

附图 1－2　诺氟沙星的 HRMS 谱图（ESI$^+$）

扫码"学一学"

Experiment 1　Synthesis of Norfloxacin

Experimental aim

1. Get preliminary knowledge of the process of new drug research through the synthesis of norfloxacin.

2. Learn how to select a practical process on the basis of comparison of several different synthetic routes.

3. Train the basic experimental technology of organic chemistry and practice handling skill of various reactions.

4. Learn the quality control method of intermediates in every reaction step.

Experimental principles

Norfloxacin

1 – ethyl – 6 – fluoro – 1,4 – dihydro – 4 – oxo – 7 – (1 – piperazinyl) – 3 – quindinecarboxylic acid

Norfloxacin is a white to yellow needle crystal or crystalline powder with mp. 216 ~ 220℃. It is freely soluble in acids and bases, slightly soluble in water, acetone and ethanol.

There are many preparation routesof norfloxacin based on different starting materials. However, there are only a couple of routes which could be used in the industry. The current industrial process in China is shown as follow.

Condensation of 3 – chloro – 4 – fluoro aniline (1 – 1) with diethyl – ethoxymethylenemalonate (EMME) followed by the cyclization yields ethyl 6 – fluro – 7 – chloro – 1,4 – dihydro – 4 – oxo – quinoline – 3 – carboxylate (1 – 3). The compound (1 – 3) is ethylated with ethyl bromide to give ethyl 1 – ethyl – 6 – fluro – 7 – chloro – 1,4 – dihydro – 4 – oxo – quinoline – 3 – carboxylate (1 – 4), which reacts with acetic anhydride and boric acid (AcO_3B) to form a boron chelating compound (1 – 5). The boron chelating compound (1 – 5) condenses with piperazine in DMSO and then is hydrolyzed with sodium hydroxide to yield norfloxacin.

（1–1）　　　　　　　　　　EMME →　　　　　　　　　（1–2）　　→

The reaction scheme shows the synthesis of Norfloxacin through intermediates (1-3), (1-4), (1-5), (1-6).

(1-3) →EtBr→ (1-4) →(AcO)₃B→

(1-5) →HN-piperazine-NH / DMSO→ (1-6) →(1) H⁺ (2) OH⁻→

Norfloxacin

Pre – lab preparation

1. Summarize other reagents for N – ethylation and compare their advantages and disadvantages.

2. Analyze what is the byproduct in this synthetic process and how to reduce the byproduct.

3. Give suggestion for making reasonable use of ethyl bromide.

4. In synthesis of (1 – 4), if the solution was directly diluted with water without lowing the temperature after recovering the DMF, what results would be obtained?

Knowledge point

Set – up of reaction apparatus, adding procedures of chemical reagents, condensation reaction, cyclization reaction, hydrolysis reaction, operation of recrystallization and extraction, purity test.

Experiment procedures

Ⅰ. **Synthesis of ethyl 7 – chloro – 6 – fluoro – 4 – oxo – 1 , 4 – dihydro quinoline – 3 – carboxylate(1 – 3)**

1. Materials(Table 1 – 1)

Table 1 – 1　Specification and ratio of raw materials

Materials	Specifications	Amount	Mol	Mol ratio
4 – fluoro – 3 – chloroaniline(1 – 1)	Industrial Material	15g	0. 103	1
EMME	Industrial Material	24g	0. 111	1. 07
Paraffin oil	CP	80ml		
Toluene	CP			
Acetone	CP			

2. Procedures 4 – Fluoro – 3 – chloroaniline(1 – 1) and EMME were added to a 150ml three neck flask equipped with stirrer, condenser and thermometer(Note 1). The mixture was heated to

120 ~ 130℃ and kept at this temperature for 2h with stirring. The reaction solution was then cooled to room temperature. The equipped flask was changed from refluxing to distillation. Paraffin oil was added to the mixture and heated to 260 ~ 270℃ (Note 2). The ethanol produced during the reaction was distilled out. After about 0.5h for distillation of ethanol, the reaction mixture was cooled to 60℃. The product precipitated at 60℃ was isolated by suction. The filtrating cake was washed with toluene and acetone respectively to give a gray – white color solid, which was dried with mp. 297 ~ 298℃. The reaction yield would be calculated(Note 3).

3. Notes

Note 1: This reaction was carried out under anhydrous environment and all glassware and flasks should be dried before use. Trace amount of water will cause the degradation of EMME.

Note 2: The temperature must be strictly controlled between 260 ~ 270℃. Before the reaction temperature reached 270℃, heating must be slowed down. The reaction liquid would become much thicker after reaction starting. Quick stirring is desirable to avoid over – heating.

Note 3: This reaction is a typical Gould – Jacobs reaction. The para – position of 3 – chloro is far more active than the ortho one. However, if the reaction conditions are not well controlled, more undesired byproducts were obtained.

To reduce the amount of the byproduct, more attention should be paid.

(1) Lower reaction temperatures prefer to form the byproduct(the ratio of the product and the byproduct could be 1 : 1, depending on the lowing reaction temperatures). So the reaction mixture should be quickly heated to 260℃ and be kept in 260 ~ 270℃.

(2) The yield of byproduct could be lower if more solvent are added. The relationship between the amount of solvent and the yield of product is shown as Table 1 – 2. A ratio of 3 : 1 in solvent and reaction materials was more suitable in economy.

(3) Using diphenyl ether or diphenylsulfone as the solvent could decrease the byproduct. However, both solvent are expensive for the industrial use. Paraffin oil is the better choice but it could be substituted by diesel fuel which is more economical.

Table 1 – 2　Effection of the ratio of solvent to reactant on the yield

Solvent/ Reaction materials	Product/Byproduct	Total yield
1 : 1	81.6 : 18.4	97.2
3 : 1	85.5 : 14.5	95.4
8 : 1	94.7 : 5.3	96.4

4. Questions

(1) Please write down the mechanism of Gould – Jacobs reaction, and discuss under what conditions the yield could be raised.

（2）This is apyroprocess reaction, list some bath for pyroprocess and give some points for safety attention.

II. Synthesis of ethyl 7 – chloro – 1 – ethyl – 6 – fluoro – 4 – oxo – 1,4 – dihydro – quinoline – 3 – carboxylate(1 – 4)

1. Materials(Table 1 – 3)

Table 1 – 3 Specification and ratio of raw materials

Materials	Specifications	Amount	Mol	Mol ratio
Cyclized compound(1 – 3)	Prepared in last step	25g	0. 093	1
Ethyl bromide	CP	25g	0. 229	2. 46
DMF	CP	125g		
Anhydrous potassium carbonate	CP	30. 8g	0. 223	2. 39

2. Procedures

The compound(1 – 3), anhydrous potassium carbonate and DMF were added to a 250ml four – neck flask fixed with stirrer, refluxing condenser, thermometer and addition funnel (Note 1). The reaction mixture was heated to 70℃ and ethyl bromide was added dropwise at 70 ~ 80℃ in 40 ~ 60min(Note 2). The reaction mixture was heated to 100 ~ 110℃ and maintained at 100 ~ 110℃ for 6 ~ 8h. After the reaction was complete, 70% ~ 80% of DMF was recovered under reduced pressure. The reaction mixture was cooled to 50℃ and 200ml water was added(Note 3). A solid precipitated out from the reaction solution(Note 4). The solid was filtered, washed with water, and dried to afford the crude product(Note 5), which was purified by recrystallization with ethanol (Note 6)with mp. 144 ~ 145℃. The yield was calculated.

3. Notes

Note 1: This reaction was also carried out under anhydrous condition and all glassware and flasks should be dried before use. DMF and K_2CO_3 should be freshly dried. Little water could have a big impact on the reaction yield.

Note 2: Because of the low boiling point of ethyl bromide, ethyl bromide should be added underneath the surface of the reaction mixture to avoid the loss of volatile ethyl bromide. The reaction flask should be tightly sealed.

Note 3: The temperature should be controlled about 50℃, when water was added to the reaction solution. High temperatures may result in the hydrolysis of the ester bond. However, lower temperatures would also result in the formation of the lumps, which could cause problems in the following steps.

Note 4: The cyclized compound forms equilibrium between the keto form and enolic form, causing the formation of a small amount of the O – ethyl byproduct. The O – ethyl byproduct was brought to the next step. O – ethyl byproduct to produce a main impurity, 6 – fluoro – 1,4 – dihydro – 4 – oxo – 7 – (piperazin – 1 – yl) – quinoline (in brief: decarboxylate), in norfloxacin. The amount of O – ethyl byproduct will change by the different ethylation agents, lower amount of O – ethyl byproduct was given by using ethyl bromide.

Note 5: The filtering cake should be grinned into a fine powder before washing with large amounts of water to ensure the K_2CO_3 in the cake washed out.

Note 6: Recrystallization was performed by refluxing the crude product in ethanol. The mixture composed of 1 part of the crude product and 4 parts of ethanol was heated to reflux to form a solution. The solution was cooled and some active charcoal was added to the solution, which was heated for another 10min. The hot solution was filtered and cooled to 10℃. The product crystallized from the solution and was separated with mp. 144 ~ 145℃. Some product in mother liquid could be obtained by concentration of mother liquid to half volume and crystallization in room temperature.

4. Questions

(1) Summary and compare the ethylation reagents.

(2) What is the byproduct of this reaction? How to reduce it?

(3) How to make reasonable use of ethyl bromide?

(4) What is the result, if the solution was directly diluted with water without lowing the temperature after recovering the DMF?

Ⅲ. Synthesis of boron chelating compound(1 - 5)

1. Materials(Table 1 - 4)

Table 1 - 4   Specification and ratio of the starting materials

Materials	Specifications	Amount	Mol	Mol ratio
Ethylated product(1 - 4)	Prepared in last step	10g	0.034	1
Boric acid	CP	3.3g	0.053	1.54
Acetic anhydride	CP	17g	0.167	4.9
Zinc chloride	CP	1g		
Ethanol	CP	Appropriate amount		

2. Procedures   Zinc chloride 1g, boric acid anda small amount of acetic anhydride were added to a 250ml four - neck bottle furnished with stirrer, condenser, thermometer and addition funnel (Note 1). The mixture in flask was heated to 79℃ with stirring. When the reaction took place, heating was stopped and the temperature of the reaction mixture raised to 120℃ by exothermal. The rest of acetic anhydride was added dropwise. The reaction mixture was then refluxed for 1h and cooled. The ethylated compound(1 - 4) obtained in last step was added. The reaction mixture was refluxed for 2.5h and cooled to room temperature. Water was added. The product was obtained by filtering and washing with cold ethanol to give a gray – white color solid(Note 2)with mp. 275℃ (dec.).

3. Notes

Note 1：The reaction of boric acid with acetic anhydride is

$$3Ac_2O + H_3BO_3 \longrightarrow (AcO)_3B$$

The reaction starts at 79℃. The temperature increased quickly because the reaction is exothermal. It is suggested to use 250ml four – neck bottle and heat slowly to reduce the risk of run away reaction.

Note 2：The boron chelating compound is soluble in ethanol. It is better to wash the wet filtering cake first with ice water then wash with cold ethanol.

4. Questions

(1)What is the influence between stirring fast and slowly?

(2)How many compounds are involved in the reaction system after ethyl agent is added?

Ⅳ. Synthesis of Norfloxacin

1. Materials(Table 1 – 5)

Table 1 – 5　Specification and ratio of raw materials

Materials	Specifications	Amount	Mol	Mol ratio
Chelated compound(1 – 5)	Prepared in last step	10g	0.025	1
Anhydrous piperazine	CP	8g	0.116	4.64
DMSO	CP	30g		
NaOH(10%)		20ml		
Acetic acid	CP	a. q.		

2. Procedures　The chelated compound(1 – 5)(Note 1), anhydrous piperazine and DMSO were added to a 150ml three – neck flask equipped with stirrer, refluxing condenser and thermometer. The mixture was reacted at 110℃ for 3 hours, then cooled to 90℃. 10% NaOH solution was added and the reaction mixture was refluxed for 2h(Note 2). When the reaction mixture became clear, heating was stopped. Norfloxacin is soluble in alkali media. The mixture was cooled to room temperature.

The mixture was diluted with 50ml water and neutralized with acetic acid to pH 7.2. Crude product was obtained after filtration and washing with water(Note 3).

The crude product was added to a 100ml beaker. 100ml water was added and the mixture was heated to for the dissolution of the product. After the mixture was cooled, the pH of the mixture was adjusted to pH 7 with acetic acid. A solid precipitated. The solid was collected by sucking and the wet cake was washed with water. Norfloxacin was dried with mp. 216 ~ 220℃.

3. Notes

Note 1：The 7 – Cl is activated and 6 – F is passivated in boron chelated compound(1 – 5)by enhancing the inducing effect through p – electron transfer from 4 – carbonyl oxygen to boron atom orbit, so as to selectively increase the yield of product(1 – 6)and completely prevent the formation of chloropropionate(byproduct).

Note 2：Norfloxacin is soluble in a basic solution. The reaction goes to completion when the solution is clear after adding sodium hydroxide.

Note 3：The acetate in filtering cake should be washed off completely to prevent it bringing into the final purification process.

4. Questions Which reagent or reagent system could be used to substitute DMSO?

【Characterization of Norfloxacin】

Melting point: 218 ~ 224℃.

^{1}H – NMR: Conforms(Attached figure 1 – 1).

HRMS(ESI$^+$): 320. 1055(M + H$^+$)(Attached figure 1 – 2).

HPLC purity: 99. 9%.

HPLC conditions:

Column: C18(4. 6mm × 250mm, 5μm).

Flow rate: 1. 0ml/min.

Injection volume: 10μl.

Detection wavelength: 278nm.

Mobile phase A: 0. 025mol/L Phosphoric acid(adjust to pH = 3. 0 ± 0. 1 with triethylamine) – Acetonitrile(87 : 13); Mobile phase B: Acetonitrile. Perform gradient elution according to Table 1 – 6. Ultrasonic degassing before use.

Table 1 – 6 Elution gradient

Time/min	Mobile phase A/%	Mobile phase B/%
0	100	0
10	100	0
20	50	50
30	50	50
32	100	0
42	100	0

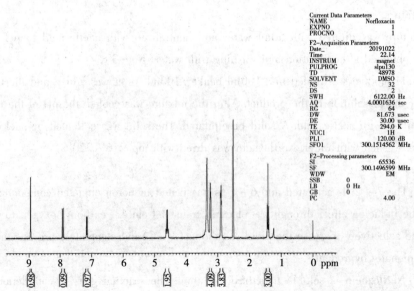

Attached figure 1 – 1 ^{1}H – NMR spectrum of norfloxacin(DMSO – d$_6$)

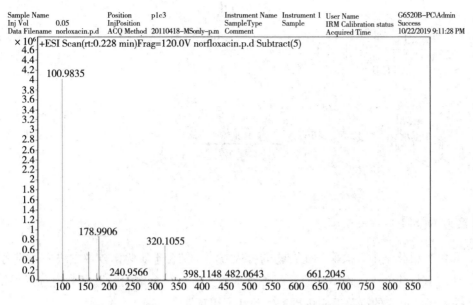

Sample Name | Position p1c3 | Instrument Name Instrument 1 | User Name G6520B-PC\Admin
Inj Vol 0.05 | InjPosition | SampleType Sample | IRM Calibration status Success
Data Filename norloxacin.p.d | ACQ Method 20110418-MSonly-p.m | Comment | Acquired Time 10/22/2019 9:11:28 PM

+ESI Scan(rt:0.228 min)Frag=120.0V norfloxacin.p.d Subtract(5)

Attached figure 1 – 2　HRMS spectrum of norfloxacin(ESI$^+$)

实验二　盐酸普鲁卡因的合成

【实验目的】

1. 通过局部麻醉药盐酸普鲁卡因的合成，学习酯化、还原等单元反应。
2. 掌握利用水和二甲苯共沸脱水的原理进行羧酸的酯化操作。
3. 掌握水溶性大的盐类用盐析法进行分离及精制的方法。

【实验原理】

盐酸普鲁卡因（procaine hydrochloride）的化学名称为2-（二乙胺基）乙基4-氨基苯甲酸酯盐酸盐，［2-（diethylamino）ethyl 4-aminobenzoate hydrochloride］。化学结构式为：

盐酸普鲁卡因为白色结晶或结晶性粉末，无臭，味微苦，随后有麻痹感。熔点155～156℃。本品在水中易溶，略溶于乙醇，微溶于三氯甲烷，不溶于乙醚。

17

$$\xrightarrow[\text{45℃，2小时}]{\text{Fe/HCl}}$$

（2-3）

$$\xrightarrow[]{\text{20\%NaOH}}$$

（2-4）

$$\xrightarrow[\text{pH 5.5}]{\text{HCl}}$$

盐酸普鲁卡因

【实验预习】

1. 预习有机化学中有关酯类化合物的合成方法，结合本实验比较各方法之间的优缺点。

2. 预习有机化学中，由硝基还原制备氨基的反应，结合本实验思考为何选择用铁粉还原以及铁粉还原反应的有关反应机制和实验注意事项。

3. 预习用硫化钠除铁以及用盐酸除去硫的原理。

4. 预习课本中有关盐酸普鲁卡因合成的原理、盐酸普鲁卡因的性质及分解产物。

5. 预习有关盐析的基本原理。

【知识点】

仪器装置，投料过程，铁粉还原硝基制备氨基，盐析的基本原理，硫化钠除铁，盐酸除硫。

【实验步骤】

（一）β-二乙胺基乙基4-硝基苯甲酸酯（硝基卡因）（2-2）的制备

1. 原料规格及配比　见表2-1。

表2-1　原料规格及配比表

原料名称	规格	用量	摩尔数	摩尔比
对硝基苯甲酸	工业用，含量＞96%，水分＜1%	20.0g	0.12	1
β-二乙胺基乙醇	CP，$d=0.88$，b. p. 163℃	14.7g	0.123	1.044
二甲苯	CP，$d=0.88$，b. p. 163℃	150ml		

2. 实验操作　在装有温度计、分水器及回流冷凝器的500ml三颈瓶中（附注1）投入对硝基苯甲酸（2-1）、β-二乙胺基乙醇、二甲苯及止爆剂，油溶加热至回流（注意控制温度，油溶温度约为180℃，内温约为145℃），共沸带水6小时（附注2）。撤去油浴，稍冷，倒入250ml锥形瓶中，放置冷却至室温，析出固体。

将上清液用倾泻法转移至分液漏斗中，用3% 盐酸水溶液提取3次（2×50ml，1×40ml），提取液与锥形瓶中的固体合并，用布氏漏斗过滤，除去未反应的对硝基苯甲酸（附注3），滤液［含硝基卡因（2-2）］，供下步还原反应使用。

3. 附注

（1）羧酸和醇之间进行的酯化反应是一个可逆反应。

$$RCOOH + R'OH \rightleftharpoons RCOOR' + H_2O$$

反应达到平衡时，生成酯的量比较少（约 65.2%），为使平衡向右移动，须向反应体系中不断加入反应原料或不断除去生成物。本反应利用二甲苯和水形成共沸混合物的原理，将生成的水不断除去，从而打破平衡，使酯化反应趋于完全。由于水的存在对反应产生不利的影响，故实验中所用的药品和仪器应事前干燥。

常用的共沸脱水体系如表 2-2 所示。

表 2-2 常用的共沸脱水体系

| 组分 A | | 组分 B | | 共沸混合物 | |
名称	沸点/℃	名称	沸点/℃	A 组分重量/%	共沸沸点/℃
水	100	苯	80.2	8.83	69.25
水	100	甲苯	110.7	13.5	84.1
水	100	二甲苯	139	35.8	92
水	100	氯苯	131.8	28.4	90.2
水	100	硝基苯	210.85	88	98.6
水	100	乙苯	136.2	33	92

（2）考虑到教学实验的需要和可能，将分水反应时间定为 6 小时，若延长反应时间收率尚可提高。

（3）对硝基苯甲酸应除尽，否则影响产品质量，回收的对硝基苯甲酸经处理后可以套用。

（二）β-二乙胺基乙基 4-氨基苯甲酸酯（普鲁卡因）（2-4）的制备

1. 原料规格及配比 见表 2-3。

表 2-3 原料规格及配比表

原料名称	规格	用量	摩尔数	摩尔比
硝基卡因盐酸溶液（2-2）	上一步自制	上步得量		
铁粉	工业还原铁粉粒度：80 目，无油污、铁锈	47g	0.83	

2. 实验操作 将上步得到的滤液转移至装有搅拌器、温度计的 500ml 三颈瓶中，搅拌下用 20% 氢氧化钠调节 pH 至 4.0~4.2，充分搅拌下，于 25℃ 分次加入经活化的铁粉（附注 1）。反应温度自动上升（附注 2），注意控制温度不要使其超过 70℃（必要时可冷却），待铁粉加毕，于 40~45℃ 保温反应 2 小时。抽滤，滤渣以少量的水洗两次，滤液以稀盐酸酸化至 pH=5。滴加饱和硫化钠溶液至 pH=7.8~8.0，沉淀反应液中的铁盐，抽滤，滤渣以少量的水洗涤二次，滤液用稀盐酸酸化至 pH=6（附注 3）。加少量活性炭于 50~60℃ 保温 10 分钟后抽滤，滤渣以少量水洗一次，将滤液冷却至 10℃ 以下，用 20% 氢氧化钠碱化至普鲁卡因全部析出为止（pH 为 9.5~10.5），过滤，抽干，得普鲁卡因，供下一步成盐用。

3. 附注

（1）铁粉活化的目的是除去其表面的铁锈，其方法为：取铁粉 47g，加水 100ml，浓盐酸 0.7ml，加热至微沸，用水倾泻法洗至近中性，置水中保存待用。

（2）该反应系放热反应，铁粉应分次加入，以免反应过于激烈，加入铁粉后温度自然上升。铁粉加毕后，待其温度降至 45℃ 进行保温反应。在反应过程铁粉参加反应后，生成绿色沉淀 $[Fe(OH)_2]$，接着变成棕色 $[Fe(OH)_3]$，然后转变为棕黑色的 Fe_3O_4。因此在反应过程中经历绿→棕→黑的颜色变化，若反应过程中，不转变为棕黑色，可能系反应尚未完全。可补加适量铁粉，继续反应一段时间。

（3）因除铁时溶液中有过量的硫化钠存在，加酸后可使其形成胶体硫，加活性炭后过滤，便可使其除去。

（三）盐酸普鲁卡因的制备

1. 原料规格与配比 见表2-4。

表2-4 原料规格与配比表

原料名称	规格	用量	摩尔数	摩尔比
普鲁卡因	自制	上步得量		1
盐酸	CP, $d=1.8$	适量		
食盐	精制品	适量		
保险粉	CP	食盐的1%		

2. 实验操作

（1）成盐 将上步所得普鲁卡因置于小烧杯中（附注1），慢慢滴加浓盐酸至 pH 5.5（附注2），加热至60℃，加精制食盐至饱和。升温至60℃，加入适量保险粉（附注3），再加热至65~70℃，趁热过滤，滤液冷却结晶，待冷至10℃以下，过滤，即得普鲁卡因粗品。

（2）精制 将上步所得粗品置洁净的小烧杯中，滴加蒸馏水至维持在70℃时恰好溶解，加入适量的保险粉，于70℃保温反应10分钟，趁热过滤，滤液自然冷却。当有结晶析出时，外用冰浴冷却，使结晶完全。过滤，滤滤并用少量冷乙醇洗涤二次，在红外灯下干燥得盐酸普鲁卡因成品，产量 8~10g，mp. 153~157℃，总收率为 24.5%~30.7%（以对硝基苯甲酸计）。

3. 附注

（1）盐酸普鲁卡因水溶性很大，所用仪器必须干燥，用水量应严格控制，否则影响收率。

（2）严格控制 pH=5.5，以免芳氨基成盐。

（3）保险粉为强还原剂，可防止芳氨基氧化，同时可除去有色杂质，以保证产品色泽洁白；若用量过多，则成品含硫量不合格。

4. 思考题

（1）在盐酸普鲁卡因制备中为何用对硝基苯甲酸为原料先酯化，然后再进行还原，能否反之先还原后酯化，即用对氨基苯甲酸为原料进行酯化，为什么？

（2）酯化反应中，为何加入二甲苯作溶剂？

（3）酯化反应结束后，放冷除去的固体是什么？为什么要除去？

（4）在铁粉还原过程中，为什么会发生颜色变化？说出其反应机制。

（5）还原反应结束，为什么要加入硫化钠？

（6）在盐酸普鲁卡因成盐和精制时，为什么要加入保险粉？解释其原理。

【盐酸普鲁卡因的结构表征】

熔点：155~156℃。

^{1}H-NMR：结构正确（附图2-1）。

HRMS（ESI$^+$）：237.1280（M+H$^+$）（附图2-2）。

HPLC 测试的色谱条件：

色谱柱：Xtimate™ C18（4.6μm×150mm，5μm）。

流速：1ml/min。

进样量：10μl。

检测波长：290nm。

柱温：30℃。

流动相：缓冲液：甲醇＝68∶32。缓冲液：以 0.1% 庚烷磺酸钠与 0.05mol/L 磷酸二氢钾溶液（用磷酸调节 pH 3.0）－甲醇＝68∶32 为流动相，均用 0.45μm 滤膜过滤。使用前需超声脱气。

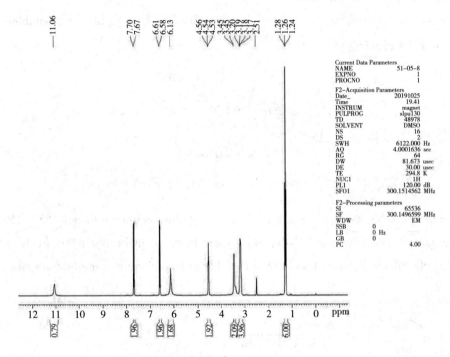

附图 2 − 1　盐酸普鲁卡因的 ^1H − NMR 谱图（DMSO − d_6）

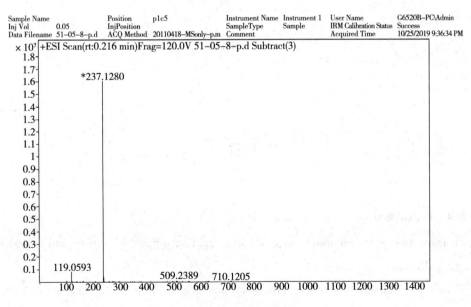

附图 2 − 2　盐酸普鲁卡因的 HRMS 谱图（ESI$^+$）

扫码"学一学"

Experiment 2　　Synthesis of Procaine Hydrochloride

Experimental aim

1. Learn the esterification and reduction reactions through the synthesis of Procaine hydrochloride.

2. Train the operation of the esterification of the carboxylic acid with the alcohol through azeotropic removal of water with xylene.

3. Practice the method for the separation and purification of the highly water soluble salts.

Experimental principles

Procaine hydrochloride

2 – (diethylamino) ethyl 4 – aminobenzoate hydrochloride

Procaine hydrochloride is a white crystal or a crystalline powder with mp. $155 \sim 156 \,^\circ\!C$. It is odorless, slightly bitter taste and subsequently numb. Procaine hydrochloride is freely soluble in water, sparingly soluble in ethanol and slightly soluble in chloroform and insoluble in ether.

（2–1）　　HO　　Xylene, 145℃, 6h　　（2–2）

Fe/HCl
45℃, 2h　　（2–3）　　20%NaOH

（2–4）　　HCl
pH 5.5　　Procaine Hydrochloride

Pre – lab preparation

1. Summary the ester preparation methods from acid in organic chemistry and compare their advantages and disadvantages.

2. Review the reduction reaction of nitro group to amino group in organic chemistry. Analyze the reason why iron powder reduction was chosen in this experiment and list the reaction mechanism and

experimental precautions.

3. Preview the principle of removing iron with sodium sulfide and sulfur with hydrochloric acid.

4. Preview the principle of procaine hydrochloride synthesis, the properties and decomposition products of procaine hydrochloride in the textbook.

5. Preview the basic principle of salting out.

Knowledge points

Set – up of reaction apparatus, reduction of nitro group by iron powder, basic principle of salting out; removing iron by sodium sulfide.

Experiment procedures

I. Preparation of β – diethylaminoethyl 4 – nitro – benzoate(Nitrocaine)(2 – 2)

1. Materials(Table 2 – 1)

Table 2 – 1 Specification and ratio of raw materials

Materials	Specifications	Amount	Mol	Molar ratio
p – nitrobenzoic acid(2 – 1)	Industrial reagent, content > 96%, water < 1%	20.0g	0.12	1
β – diethylaminoethanol	CP, d = 0.88, bp. 163℃	14.7g	0.123	1.044
Xylene	CP, d = 0.88, bp. 163℃	150ml		

2. Procedures To a 500ml three – neck flask equipped with a 250℃ thermometer, a water trap attached with a condenser, and an addition funnel(Note 1), p – nitrobenzoic acid(2 – 1), β – diethylaminoethanol, xylene and zeolite were added. The mixture was then heated with the oil bath to reflux. The reaction temperature was controlled at about 145℃ and the oil bath at 180℃. The reaction solution was refluxed for 6 hours(Note 2) and the water produced in the reaction was removed to water trap by azeotropic refluxation. Then the mixture was cooled and transferred to a 250ml rlenmeyer flask. The mixture was further cooled to room temperature to give the mixture of slurry.

The slurry was settled and the top clear solution was transferred to the separating funnel by decantation. The solution was extracted with 3% aqueous hydrochloric acid three times(2 × 50ml and 1 × 40ml). The extracts were combined with the solid in the erlenmeyer flask and filtered to remove the unreacted p – nitrobenzoic acid(Note 3). The filtrate containing(2 – 2) could be directly used in the next step without further purification.

3. Notes

Note 1: The esterification of the carboxylic acid with the alcohol is reversible. There is an equilibrium in which the amount of the ester produced in 65.2%.

$$RCOOH + R'OH \rightleftharpoons RCOOR' + H_2O$$

To make the reaction equilibrium shift to the product side(the right hand of the equilibrium), either one of the starting materials was more added in the left side or one of the products was removed in the right side. Based on the fact that water and xylene could form an azeotropic mixture, the water generated from the reaction was azeotropically removed from the reaction system to break the equilibrium and forced the reaction to completion. Since the existence of the water is unfavorable for the reaction, all reagents and the equipments should be dried before use.

The commonazeotropic mixtures are as Table 2 – 2.

Table 2 – 2 Commoazeotropic mixtures

Component A		Component B		Mixtures	
Name	bp/℃	Name	bp/℃	Weight of A/%	Azeotropic point/℃
Water	100	Benzene	80. 2	8. 83	69. 25
Water	100	Methyl benzene	110. 7	13. 5	84. 1
Water	100	Dimethyl benzene	139	35. 8	92
Water	100	Chlorobenzene	131. 8	28. 4	90. 2
Water	100	Nitro – benzene	210. 85	88	98. 6
Water	100	Ethylbenzene	136. 2	33	92

Note 2: The yield was little increased if the reaction time was prolonged more than 6 hours.

Note 3: The p – nitrobenzoic acid should be removed completely. Otherwise, it could affect the quality of the product. The recovered p – nitrobenzoic acid could also be reused.

Ⅱ. Preparation of 2 – diethylaminoethanol 4 – aminobenzoic acid ester(Procaine)(2 – 4)

1. Materials(Table 2 – 3)

Table 2 – 3 Specification and ratio of raw materials

Materials	Specifications	Amount	Mol	Mol ratio
Nitrocaine(2 – 2) Hydrochloride solution	Prepared in the last step	Directly used		
Iron powder	Industrial grade iron powder, 80 mesh, no oil or rust	47g	0. 83	

2. Procedures To a 500ml three – neck flask equipped with a brush peddler, a thermometer and an addition funnel, the filtrating solution obtained from the last step was transferred. Then the pH value of the solution was adjusted to 4. 0 ~ 4. 2 with 20% sodium hydroxide solution under stirring. The reaction mixture was vigorously stirred and the activated iron powder in portions was added at 25℃ (Note 1). The temperature went up gradually after the iron powder was added(Note 2). It needs to be very careful to control the temperature below 70℃. Cooling was required when necessary. After adding the iron powder, the reaction mixture was kept at 40 ~ 45℃ for 2 hours.

The reaction mixture was filtered. The filtering residue was washed twice with small amounts of water. The filtrate liquid was acidified by a dilute hydrochloric acid solution to pH 5. To the solution, the saturated sodium sulfide solution was addeddropwise to adjust pH to 7. 8 ~ 8. 0. The ferrous ion in the solution became ferrous sulfide to deposit. The precipitate was filtered and washed twice with a small amount of water. The filtrate solution was then acidified by dilute hydrochloric acid to pH 6(Note 3).

Active charcoal was added and the resulting slurry was kept at 50 ~ 60℃ for 10 minutes. The slurry was filtered and the charcoal cake was washed twice with small amounts of water. The combined filtrate solution was cooled below 10℃ and basified with 20% sodium hydroxide solution to deposit procaine completely on pH 9.5~10.5. The precipitated procaine was collected and dried for using in the next step.

3. Notes

Note 1:The iron powder should be activated to remove the rust layer on the iron surface. Water 100ml and concentrated hydrochloric acid 0.7ml were added to iron powder 47g. The mixture was heated to light boiling. Then the above acidic water solution was decanted and the iron powder was washed with water for several times by decantation until the pH value of the wash solution is neutral. The activated iron powder was kept in the water for the future immediate use.

Note 2:Since the reaction is exothermal, the iron powder should be added in small portions for several times to avoid more intensive heat generation in the reaction. After addition of iron powder, the reaction should be maintained below 45℃. During the reduction, the color of reaction system changed from green[$Fe(OH)_2$] to brown[$Fe(OH)_3$], then to black-brown[Fe_3O_4]. If the color of reaction system did not become black-brown at the end, it indicated that the reaction was not complete. More iron powder was added and the reaction was continued for more time.

Note 3:Because excess amount of sodium sulfide was used to remove the iron ions in the reaction solution, dilute hydrochloric acid was added to make excess sodium sulfide form the gel sulfur, which was removed by filtering with activated charcoal.

Ⅲ. Preparation of procaine hydrochloride

1. Materials(Table 2-4)

Table 2-4　Specification and ratio of raw materials

Materials	Specifications	Amount	Mol	Molar ratio
Procaine	Prepared in the last step	Directly used		1
Hydrochloric acid	CP, $d=1.8$	Appropriate amount		
Salt	Refine product	Appropriate amoun		
Sodium hydrosulfite	CP	1% of the salt		

2. Procedures

(1)Salt formation　Procaine(2-4)prepared last step was placed in a small beaker(Note 1), concentrated hydrochloric acid was added slowly to adjust the pH to 5.5(Note 2). The mixture was heated on the water bath to 60℃. Fine NaCl was added to the solution to saturation. An appropriate amount of sodium hydrosulfite was then added(Note 3).

The solution was heated to 65~70℃, and filtered when it was hot. The filtrate was cooled to the temperature below 10℃. The product crystallized out and the resulting slurry was filtered. The crude product of procaine hydrochloride was obtained.

(2)Recrystallization of the crude product　The crude product was transferred to a clean small beaker. An appropriate amount of distilled water was added just to give a clear solution at 70℃. An appropriate amount of sodium hydrosulfite was added and the mixture was kept at 70℃ for 10 minutes. The hot solution was filtered and the filtrating liquid was cooled slowly. When the product crystals were formed, the solution was cooled with an ice bath for the complete crystallization of the product.

The product crystals were collected and washed twice with cold ethanol. The product was dried under heat of the infrared light and weighted. The product has a melting point of $153 \sim 157$℃ and the overall yield was about 24.5% ~30.7% (calculated from p – nitrobenzoic acid).

3. Notes

Note 1: Procaine hydrochloride is water soluble and the reaction should be carried out under anhydrous conditions. All the equipments must be dried before using.

Note 2: Keeping the pH value at 5.5 is very important. Otherwise, the aromatic amine will be changed to the HCl salt form.

Note 3: Sodium hydrosulfite is a strong reducing agent to prevent the oxidation of the aromatic amine and reduce the color impurities to ensure the product as a pure white solid. Appropriate amount of sodium hydrosulfite was enough because the excess of sodium hydrosulfite might result in higher contents of sulfur in product.

4. Questions

(1) In this experiment, procaine was synthesized from p – nitrobenzoic acid through esterification and then reduction. Wether would the order be revised, p – aminobenzoic acid was used to esterification? Why?

(2) In the esterification reaction, why should xylene be used as solvent?

(3) What is the solid that is removed by cooling after the esterification reaction? Why should it be removed?

(4) Why does the color change occur during the reduction by iron powder reduction process? Explain the phenomenon by the reaction mechanism.

(5) Why should we add sodium sulfide after reduction reaction?

(6) Why should we add sodium hydrosulfite during the salt forming and the purification of procaine hydrochloride?

【Characterization of Procaine hydrochloride】

Melting point: $155 \sim 156$℃.

^{1}H – NMR(300 MHz, DMSO): Conforms(Attached figure 2 – 1).

HRMS(ESI$^+$): 237.1280(M + H$^+$)(Attached figure 2 – 2).

HPLC conditions:

Column: Xtimate^{TM} C18(4.6mm × 150mm, 5μm).

Flow rate: 1ml/min.

Injection volume: 10μl.

Detection wavelength: 290nm.

Column temperature: 30℃.

Mobile phase: Buffer: Methanol = 68 : 32. Buffer: 0.1% sodium heptanesulfonate and 0.05mol/L potassium dihydrogen phosphate solution(adjust to pH = 3.0 ±0.1 with phosphoric acid).

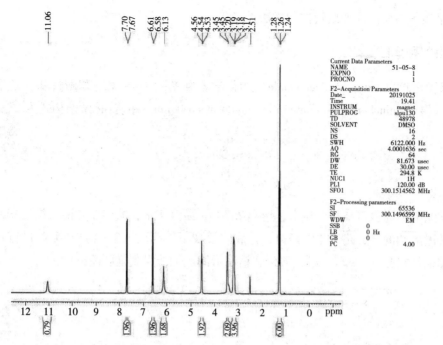

Attached figure 2 – 1 ^1H – NMR spectrum of procaine hydrochloride (DMSO – d_6)

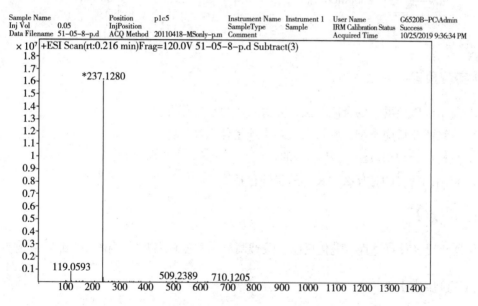

Attached figure 2 – 2 HRMS spectrum of procaine hydrochloride (ESI$^+$)

实验三 磺胺醋酰钠的合成

【实验目的】

1. 通过对磺胺醋酰钠合成工艺的研究，使学生对药物合成过程有一个基本认识。

2. 通过对磺胺醋酰钠合成路线的比较，使学生掌握选择实际生产工艺的几个基本要求。

3. 通过实际操作，熟悉各类反应特点、机制、操作要求、反应终点的控制等，进一步巩固有机化学实验的基本操作，领会掌握理论知识。

扫码"学一学"

4. 掌握各步中间体的质量控制方法。

【实验原理】

磺胺醋酰钠（sodium sulfacetamide）的化学名为 N-［（4-氨基苯磺酰基）乙酰胺单钠盐，［N-（4-aminobenzenesulfonyl）acetamide monosodium salt］。化学结构式为：

磺胺醋酰钠为白色结晶性粉末，熔点 257℃。易溶于水，略溶于乙醇，微溶于丙酮。

磺胺醋酰钠的合成路线非常经典，合成路线如下。磺胺（3-1）与醋酐进行乙酰化得到磺胺醋酰钠粗品（3-2），经过酸化和精制再制成钠盐得到磺胺醋酰钠。

【实验预习】

1. 总结磺胺醋酰钠的合成方法，并对其优缺点进行评价。
2. 总结酰化反应类型，各自的注意事项是什么？
3. 分析后处理的方法，pH 调节的作用。
4. 重结晶的目的是什么？具体的步骤包括哪些？

【知识点】

仪器装置，投料过程，酰化反应，酸碱调节，酸度解离常数（pK_a），纯度检查。

【实验步骤】

（一）磺胺醋酰钠粗品（3-2）的制备

1. 原料规格及配比 见表 3-1。

表 3-1 原料规格及配比表

原料名称	规格	用量	摩尔数	摩尔比
磺胺（3-1）	工业品	17.2g	0.10	1
醋酐	CP	13.6ml	0.14	1.4
22.5% NaOH 水溶液	自配	22.0ml	0.11	1.1
77.0% NaOH 水溶液	自配	12.5ml	0.19	1.9

2. 实验操作 在装有搅拌器、温度计和回流冷凝管的三颈瓶中投入磺胺及氢氧化钠溶液（22.5%），搅拌下加热至50℃左右，待物料溶解后，滴加醋酐3.6ml，5分钟后缓慢滴

28

加77%的氢氧化钠液2.5ml（附注1），并保持反应液pH在12~13之间，随后每隔5分钟交替滴加醋酐及氢氧化钠液，每次2ml（附注2），加料期间反应温度维持在50~55℃及pH 12~13（附注3）。加料毕，继续保温搅拌反应30分钟。

3. 附注

（1）本实验中使用氢氧化钠溶液有多种不同的浓度，在实验中切勿用错。否则会导致实验失败。

（2）滴加醋酐和氢氧化钠溶液是交替进行的，每滴完一种溶液后，让其反应5分钟后，再滴入另一种溶液。滴加是用玻璃吸管加入，滴加速度以液滴逐滴滴下为宜。

（3）反应中保持反应液pH在12~13之间很重要，否则收率将会降低。

4. 思考题

（1）反应过程中，调节溶液的pH在12~13是非常重要的。若碱性过强或碱性过弱，会产生何种结果？

（2）试分析醋酐的作用，有没有其他试剂可以替换？

（二）磺胺醋酰（3-3）的制备

1. 原料规格及配比 见表3-2。

表3-2 原料规格及配比表

原料名称	规格	用量
磺胺醋酰钠粗品（3-2）	上步自制	
水	CP	20ml
浓盐酸	CP	
10% HCl 水溶液	自配	
40% NaOH 水溶液	自配	

2. 实验操作 将反应液转入100ml烧杯中，加水20ml稀释。用浓盐酸调pH至7，于冰浴中放置1~2小时，冷却析出固体。抽滤固体，用适量冰水洗涤（附注1）。

洗液与滤液合并后用浓盐酸调pH 4~5，滤取沉淀压干（附注2）。沉淀用3倍量的10%盐酸溶解，放置30分钟，抽滤除去不溶物（附注3），滤液加少量活性炭室温脱色后，用40%氢氧化钠溶液调pH至5析出磺胺醋酰，抽滤，于红外灯下干燥得10g，mp. 179~184℃（附注4）。如熔点不合格，可用热水（1:15）精制。

3. 附注

（1）在pH 7时析出的固体不是产物，应弃去。产物在滤液中，切勿搞错。

（2）该固体是产品磺胺醋酰和副产品磺胺双醋酰的混合物。

（3）由于磺胺醋酰呈弱酸性，不能溶于酸性溶液中。

（4）在本实验中，溶液pH的调节是反应能否成功的关键，应小心注意，否则实验会失败或收率降低。

4. 思考题

（1）试分析pKa与pH的关系，并解释利用不同pH进行分离的原理。

（2）pH=7、pH=5时析出的固体是什么？10%盐酸中的不溶物是什么？

（三）磺胺醋酰钠的制备

1. 原料规格及配比 见表3-3。

表3-3　原料规格及配比表

原料名称	规格	用量
磺胺醋酰（3-3）	上步自制	
20% NaOH 水溶液	自制	

2. 实验操作　将上一步所得的磺胺醋酰（3-3）投入 50ml 烧杯中，滴加少量水润湿（<0.5ml）（附注1）。于水浴上加热至 90℃，滴加 20% 氢氧化钠至恰好溶解，溶液 pH 为 7~8，趁热抽滤，滤液转至小烧杯中放冷析出结晶（附注2），抽滤，干燥，得磺胺醋酰钠 9g。

3. 附注

（1）加入水的量以使磺胺醋酰略湿即可。0.5ml 较难掌握，可适当多加入一些（1ml 左右），在析晶时再蒸发去一些水分。

（2）此步须趁热过滤，漏斗应先预热。若滤液放置后较难析出结晶，可置电炉上略加热，使其挥发去一些水分，再放冷析晶。

4. 思考题　磺胺类药物有哪些理化性质? 在本实验中，如何利用这些性质进行产品纯化的?

【磺胺醋酰的结构表征】

熔点：257℃。

^{1}H-NMR：结构正确（附图3-1）。

MS（EI$^+$）：214.24（附图3-2）。

HPLC 纯度：99.5%。

HPLC 测试的色谱条件：

色谱柱：十八烷基硅烷键合硅胶（4.6mm×150mm，5μm）。

流速：1.0ml/min。

进样量：10μl。

检测波长：245nm。

流动相：甲醇（加 0.1% 甲酸）：水 = 1:1。使用前需超声脱气。

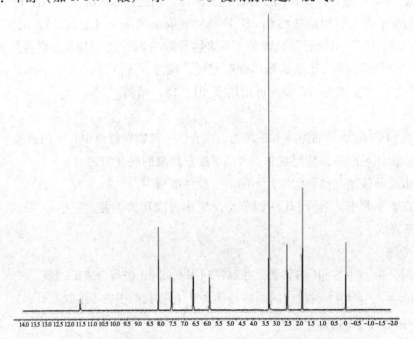

附图3-1　磺胺醋酰的 ^{1}H-NMR 谱图（DMSO-d$_6$）

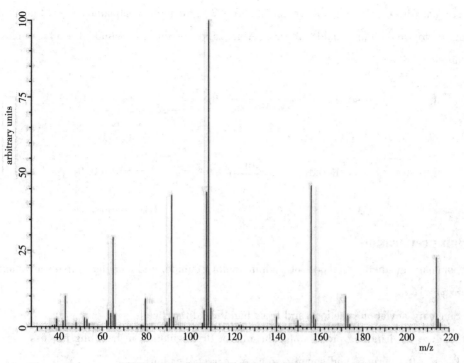

附图 3 – 2　磺胺醋酰的 HRMS 谱图（EI⁺）

Experiment 3　Synthesis of Sodium Sulfacetamide

扫码"学一学"

Experimental aim

1. Get preliminary knowledge of the process of drug synthesis through the synthesis of sodium sulfacetamide.

2. Learn how to select a practical process on the basis of comparison of several different synthetic routes.

3. Train the basic experimental technology of organic chemistry and practice handling skill of various reactions.

4. Learn the quality control method of intermediates in every reaction step.

Experimental principles

Sodium sulfacetamide

N – (4 – aminobenzenesulfonyl) acetamide monosodium salt

Sodium sulfacetamide is a white crystalline powder with mp. 257℃. It is freely soluble in water, sparingly soluble in ethanol, and slightly soluble in acetone.

The preparation route of sodium sulfacetamide is shown as follow. Sulfanilamide (3 – 1) reacted with acetic anhydride to obtain the compound（3－2）, then the compound（3－2）is purified by adjusting pH to yield sulfacetamide（3－3）. Alkalization of the compound（3－3）to yield sodium sulfacetamide.

$$H_2N \text{—} \langle \rangle \text{—} SO_2NH_2 \xrightarrow[\text{NaOH}]{(CH_3CO)_2O} H_2N \text{—} \langle \rangle \text{—} SO_2N\text{-}COCH_3 \xrightarrow{H^+}$$

（3–1）

$$\underset{Na}{|}$$

（3–2）

$$H_2N \text{—} \langle \rangle \text{—} SO_2NHCOCH_3 \xrightarrow{\text{NaOH}} H_2N \text{—} \langle \rangle \text{—} SO_2N\text{-}COCH_3$$

（3–3）

$$\underset{Na}{|}$$

Sodium sulfacetamide

Pre－lab preparation

1. Summary synthetic methods of sodium sulfacetamide and compare their advantages and disadvantages.

2. Summary acylation reactions and their handling difference.

3. Analyze the handling process and the role of pH regulation in handling process.

4. Discuss the purpose and specific steps of recrystallization.

Knowledge point

Set－up of reaction apparatus, acylation reaction, recrystallization, acid－base adjustment, purity test.

Experiment procedures

Ⅰ. Synthesis of crude Sodium Sulfacetamide（3－2）

1. Materials（Table 3－1）

Table 3－1　Specification and ratio of raw materials

Materials	Specifications	Amount	Mol	Mol ratio
Sulfanilamide（3－1）	Industral purity	17.2g	0.10	1
Acetic anhydride	CP	13.6ml	0.14	1.4
22.5% sodium hydroxide solution	Self－prepared	22.0ml	0.11	1.1
77% sodium hydroxide solution	Self－prepared	12.5ml	0.19	1.9

2. Procedures　To a 60ml four－necked flask equipped with a stirrer, a refluxing condenser and a thermometer, sulfanilamide（3－1）17.2g and 22.5% sodium hydroxide aqueous solution 22ml are added. The mixture reacted at 50℃ in a water bath. After the sulfanilamide dissolved, acetic anhydride 3.6ml is added by dropwise. After 5 minutes, 77% sodium hydroxide aqueous solution 2.5ml is added in dropwise（Note 1）. Then acetic anhydride and 77% sodium hydroxide aqueous solution are added by dropwise every 5 minutes alternately, each one 2ml every time（Note 2）. The pH of the solution should be kept between 12 to 13（Note 3）and the temperature should be maintained between 50℃ to 55℃ during addition of acetic anhydride and sodium hydroxide aqueous solution. After addition of acetic anhydride and sodium hydroxide aqueous solution, the reaction mixture is stirred between 50℃ to 55℃ for another 30 minutes.

3. Notes

Notes 1：There are many different concentrations of sodium hydroxide solution used in this experiment. It would be careful for operation, otherwise the experiment will be unsuccessful

Notes 2：Acetic anhydride and 77% sodium hydroxide aqueous solution should be added every 5 minutes alternately. After a kind of solution is added, let it react for 5 minutes and then another solution is added. The solution should be added drop by drop.

Notes 3：It is important to keep the pH of the solution between 12 and 13, otherwise the reaction yield will lower.

4. Questions

（1）It is important to keep the pH of the solution between 12 and 13. What are the results, if the pH of the solution is more basic or less basic?

（2）Please explain the effect of acetic anhydride, and try to choose another reagent to instead of it.

Ⅱ. Synthesis of Sulfacetamide(3 −3)

1. Materials(Table 3 −2)

Table 3 −2　Specification and ratio of raw materials

Materials	Specifications	Amount
CrudeSodium Sulfacetamide(3 −2)	Self − prepared	
Water	CP	20ml
Hydrochloric acid	CP	
10% HCl solution	Self − prepared	
40% NaOH solution	Self − prepared	

2. Procedures The reaction mixture from last step is poured into a 100ml beaker and water 20ml is added. The pH of the solution is adjusted to 7 with concentrated hydrochloric acid. The beaker is put in the ice − water bath for about 1 ~ 2 hours and a precipitate is produced. The solid products are collected by suction and washed with a little of ice water. (Note 1).

The above filtrating solution and washing liquid are combined, transferred to a beaker and adjusted to pH 4 ~ 5 with concentrated hydrochloric acid. A solid is deposited and collected by suction(Note 2). The solid is put into a beaker and dissolved with 3 times of 10% hydrochloric acid. The solution is settled for 30 minutes and the undissolved solid is removed by filtration(Note 3). The filtering liquid is adjusted to pH 5 with 40% sodium hydroxide aqueous solution. Sulfacetamide precipitates from the solution and is collected by suction with mp. 179 ~ 184℃ (Note 4).

3. Notes

Note 1：The solid which is precipitated at pH =7 is not the product. It is unreacted sulfanilamide. The product exists in filtrate.

Note 2：The solid is a mixture of sulfacetamide product and sulfdiacetamide byproduct.

Note 3：Because sulfacetamide shows weak acidity, it can not dissolve in the acidic solution.

Note 4：During this experiment, it is important to adjust the pH of the solution carefully.

Otherwise the reaction yield will be reduced and even the experiment will be failure.

4. Questions

(1) Analysis the relationship of pK_a and pH, and explain the principles of separation product and by products in different pH.

(2) What is the solid obtained at pH = 7 and pH = 5 respectively? What is the undissolved solid in 10% hydrochloric acid?

Ⅲ. Synthesis of Sodium Sulfacetamide

1. Materials(Table 3 - 3)

Table 3 - 3　Specification and ratio of raw materials

Materials	Specifications	Amount	Mol	Mol ratio
Sulfacetamide(3 - 3)	Self - prepared			
20% Sodium hydroxide solution	Self - prepared			

2. Procedures　The sulfacetamide(3 - 3) obtained in the last step is put into a 50ml beaker and is just wet by a little water(<0. 5ml) (Note 1). The beaker is heated to 90℃ in the water - bath, then 20% sodium hydroxide aqueous solution is added in drops until sulfacetamide is just dissolved. The pH of solution should be kept between 7 ~ 8. The solution is then filtrated while the solution is hot(Note 2). The filtrating liquid is removed to a beaker and cooled, then a solid is precipitated. The precipitated solid 9g is collected by suction and dried. This solid is sulfacetamide sodium.

3. Notes

Note 1: Be sure not to add too much water, 1ml water is acceptable to just wet sulfacetamide. Some water could be evaporated during crystal formation process if necessary.

Note 2: The funnel should be warmed - up before filtrating. If no solid come out after a long time, the solution in the beaker can be heated to evaporate some water, then the solid may come out after the solution is cooled.

4. Questions　What are the physical and chemical features of sulfacetamide? How to purify the compound by using these features?

【Characterization of Sulfacetamide】

Melting point: 257℃.

^1H – NMR: Conforms(Attached figure 3 - 1).

MS(EI): 214. 24(Attached figure 3 - 2).

HPLC purity: 99. 5%.

HPLC conditions:

Column: C18(4. 6mm × 150mm, 5μm).

Flow rate: 1. 0ml/min.

Injection volume: 10μl.

Detection wavelength：245nm.

Mobile phase：Methanol（with 0.1% formic acid）– Water（1 ： 1）. Ultrasonic degassing before use.

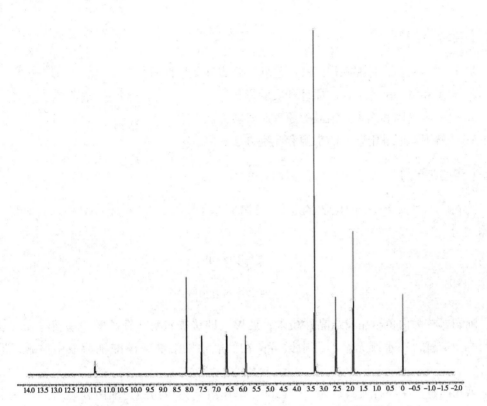

Attached figure 3 – 1　¹H – NMR spectrum of sulfacetamide（DMSO – d₆）

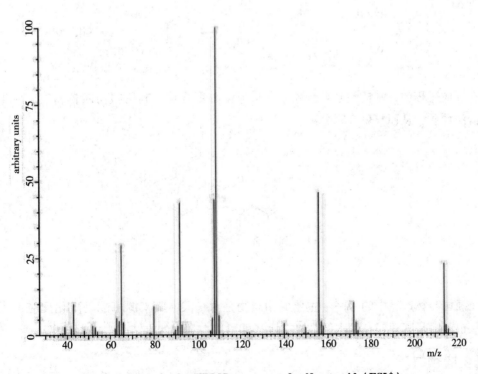

Attached figure 3 – 2　HRMS spectrum of sulfacetamide（ESI⁺）

扫码"学一学"

实验四　阿司匹林（乙酰水杨酸）的合成

【实验目的】

1. 通过本实验，掌握阿司匹林的性状、特点和化学性质。
2. 熟悉和掌握酯化反应的原理和实验操作。
3. 进一步巩固和熟悉重结晶的原理和实验方法。
4. 了解阿司匹林中杂质的来源和鉴别方法。

【实验原理】

阿司匹林（aspirin）的化学名为 2 - 乙酰氧基苯甲酸，[2 - acetoxybenzoic acid]。化学结构式为：

阿司匹林为白色结晶或结晶性粉末；遇湿气即缓缓水解。在乙醇中易溶，在三氯甲烷或乙醚中溶解，在水或无水乙醚中微溶；在氢氧化钠溶液或碳酸钠溶液中溶解，但同时分解。

阿司匹林的主要合成路线为：以乙酸乙酯作溶剂，水杨酸与醋酐在硫酸的催化下发生酯化反应，得到乙酰水杨酸（阿司匹林）粗品，然后经纯化得到阿司匹林精品。

水杨酸　　　　　　　　　　　　　　　　　　　阿司匹林

在反应过程中，水杨酸会自身缩合，形成一种聚合物。利用阿司匹林和碱反应生成水溶性盐的性质，从而与聚合物分离。

聚合物

在阿司匹林产品中的另一个主要的副产物是水杨酸，其来源可能是酰化反应不完全的原料，也可能是阿司匹林的水解产物。水杨酸可以在最后的重结晶中加以分离。

【实验预习】

1. 在阿司匹林的合成过程中，要加入少量的浓硫酸，其作用是什么？除硫酸外，是否可以用其他酸代替？

2.《中国药典》规定，成品阿司匹林中要检测水杨酸的量，为什么？本实验中采用什么方法来测定水杨酸，试简述其基本原理。

【知识点】

仪器装置，投料过程，酯化反应，重结晶，纯度检查，TLC 操作。

【实验步骤】

1. 原料规格及配比　见表 4-1。

表 4-1　原料规格及配比表

原料名称	规格	用量	摩尔数	摩尔比
水杨酸	药用	10.0g	0.075	1
醋酐	CP	25ml	0.25	3.3
乙酸乙酯	CP	10~15ml		
浓硫酸	CP	25 滴（约 1.5ml）		

2. 实验操作　在装有搅拌器、回流冷凝管和温度计的 500ml 的三颈瓶中，放入水杨酸 10.0g、醋酐 25.0ml 和沸石，然后用滴管加入浓硫酸，搅拌下使水杨酸溶解，并慢慢加热至 85~95℃（附注 1），维持温度 10 分钟。停止加热，将三颈瓶从热源上取下，使其慢慢冷却至室温。在冷却过程中，阿司匹林渐渐从溶液中析出（附注 2）。在冷到室温结晶形成后，加入水 250ml（附注 3）；并将该溶液放入冰浴中冷却。待充分冷却后，大量固体析出，抽滤得到固体，冰水洗涤，并尽量压紧抽干，得到阿司匹林粗品。

将阿司匹林粗品放在 150ml 烧杯中，边搅拌边滴加饱和的碳酸氢钠水溶液 125ml（附注 4）。在滴加碳酸氢钠水溶液时，产生大量的二氧化碳气泡并从溶液中溢出，边加边搅拌直至没有二氧化碳放出为止（无气泡放出，嘶嘶声停止）。若有不溶的固体存在，真空抽滤，除去不溶物并用少量水洗涤。另取 150ml 烧杯一只，放入浓盐酸 17.5ml 和水 50ml，将得到的滤液慢慢地分多次倒入烧杯中，边倒边搅拌。阿司匹林从溶液中析出（附注 5）。将烧杯放入冰浴中冷却，抽滤固体，并用冷水洗涤，抽紧压干固体，得阿司匹林粗品，熔点 135~136℃。

将所得的阿司匹林放入 25ml 锥形瓶中，加入少量的热的醋酸乙酯（不超过 15ml）和沸石 2 粒，在蒸汽浴上缓缓地不断地加热直至固体溶解，冷却至室温，或用冰浴冷却（附注 6），阿司匹林渐渐析出，抽滤得到阿司匹林精品（附注 7）。

3. 附注

（1）加热的热源可以是蒸汽浴、电加热套、电热板，也可以是烧杯加水的水浴。若加热的介质为水时，要注意，不要让水蒸气进入锥形瓶中，以防止酸酐和生成的阿司匹林水解。

（2）倘若在冷却过程中阿司匹林没有从反应液中析出，可用玻璃棒或不锈钢刮勺，轻轻摩擦锥形瓶的内壁，也可同时将锥形瓶放入冰浴中冷却促使结晶生成。

（3）加水时要注意，一定要等结晶充分形成后才能加入。加水时要慢慢加入，并有放热现象，甚至会使溶液沸腾。操作中会产生醋酸蒸气，必须小心，最好在通风橱中进行。

（4）当碳酸氢钠水溶液加到阿司匹林中时，会产生大量的气泡，注意分批少量地加入，一边加一边搅拌，以防气泡产生过多引起溶液外溢。

（5）如果将滤液加入盐酸后，仍没有固体析出，测一下溶液的 pH 是否呈酸性，如果不是再补加盐酸至溶液 pH 2 左右，会有固体析出。

（6）此时应有阿司匹林从醋酸乙酯中析出。若没有固体析出，可加热将醋酸乙酯挥发掉一些，再冷却，重复操作。

（7）阿司匹林纯度可用下列方法检查：取两根干净试管，分别放入少量的水杨酸和阿司匹林精品。加入乙醇各 1ml，使固体溶解。然后分别在每根试管中加入几滴 10% $FeCl_3$ 溶液，盛水杨酸的试管中有红色或紫色颜色出现，盛阿司匹林精品的试管中应是无色的。

4. 思考题 产生聚合物是合成中的主要副产物，生成的原理是什么？除聚合物外是否还会有其他可能的副产物？

【阿司匹林的结构表征】

熔点：136 ~ 140℃。

^1H – NMR：结构正确（附图 4 – 1）。

HRMS（ESI$^+$）：203.0031（M + Na$^+$）（附图 4 – 2）。

HPLC 纯度：99.9%。

HPLC 测试的色谱条件：

色谱柱：十八烷基硅烷键合硅胶（4.6mm × 250mm，5μm）。

流速：1.0ml/min。

进样量：10μl。

检测波长：303nm。

流动相：乙腈 – 四氢呋喃 – 冰醋酸 – 水（20 : 5 : 5 : 70）。使用前需超声脱气。

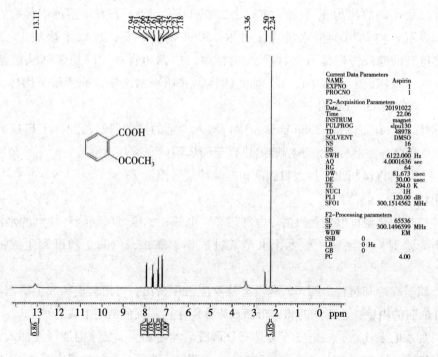

附图 4 – 1 阿司匹林的 ^1H – NMR 谱图（DMSO – d_6）

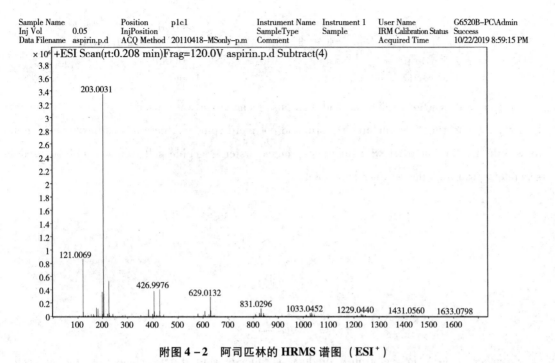

Sample Name		Position	p1c1		Instrument Name	Instrument 1	User Name	G6520B–PC\Admin
Inj Vol	0.05	InjPosition			SampleType	Sample	IRM Calibration Status	Success
Data Filename	aspirin.p.d	ACQ Method	20110418–MSonly–p.m		Comment		Acquired Time	10/22/2019 8:59:15 PM

附图 4 – 2　阿司匹林的 HRMS 谱图（ESI⁺）

Experiment 4　Synthesis of Aspirin（Acetyl Salicylic Acid）

Experimental aim

1. Learn the characters and physical and chemical properties of aspirin.

2. Review the principle and the operation of esterifaction.

3. Learn the principle and the operation of recrystallization.

4. Understand the source of the impurities in aspirin and learn how to identify them.

Experimental principles

Aspirin

2 – acetoxybenzoic acid

Aspirin is a white crystal or crystalline powder; slowly hydrolyzed in case of moisture. It is freely soluble in ethanol, soluble in chloroform or ether, and slightly soluble in water or anhydrous ether. When it is soluble in sodium hydroxide solution or sodium carbonate solution, it would be simultaneously decomposed.

The main synthesis route of aspirin is as follows: ethyl acetate is used as solvent, and salicylic acid and acetic anhydride are esterified under catalysis of sulfuric acid to obtain crude acetylsalicylic acid（aspirin）, which is then purified to obtain aspirin.

During the reaction, salicylic acid can also condensate with itself to produce a polymer byproduct. Comparing the structure of asprin and polymer byproduct, there is a carboxylic acid group in aspirin. Aspirin can react with alkali to produce water – soluble salt, which could be used to separate aspirin from the polymer byproduct.

Polymer

Another impurity in the aspirin product is salicylic acid. It may come from the unreacted material or the hydrolysis product of aspirin. The salicylic acid can be removed from aspirin by recrystallization.

Pre – lab preparation

1. Understand the effect of concentrated sulfuric acid in the preparation of aspirin. Could it be substituted by other acid?

2. Why should the content of salicylic acid in aspirin be determined? What is the method for determination of salicylic acid in this experiment?

Knowledge point

Set – up of reaction apparatus, adding procedures of chemical reagents, esterification reaction, recrystallization, purity test, TLC operation.

Experiment procedures

1. Materials(Table 4 – 1)

Table 4 – 1   Specification and ratio of raw materials

Materials	Specifications	Amount	Mol	Mol ratio
Salicylic acid	Medicinal grade	10. 0g	0. 075	1
Acetic anhydride	CP	25ml	0. 25	3. 3
Ethyl acetate	CP	10 ~ 15ml		
Concentrated sulfuric acid	CP	25 drops(about 1. 5ml)		

2. Procedures   To a 500ml three – necked flask equipped with a stirrer, refluxing condenser and a thermometer, salicylic acid 10g and acetic anhydride 25ml are added, and then the concentrated sulfuric acid is added through a burette, two pieces of zeolite are also added. The mixture with stirring is heated slowly to 85 ~ 95℃ (Note 1) and maintained for 10 minutes. After heating is stopped, the flask is taken away from the heater and cooled to room temperature slowly. During this time, Aspirin is precipitated little by little (Note 2). After the formation of the crystal, water 250ml is added and the solution is cooled with ice bath. (Note 3). When the solution is fully cooled, great amount of solid is precipitated. The solid is filtered, washed with ice water and pressed, and the crude product of aspirin is obtained.

The crude product of aspirin is put into a 150ml beaker, and saturated sodium bicarbonate aqueous solution 125ml is added with stirring (Note 4). During adding sodium bicarbonate aqueous solution, a lot of carbon dioxide bubbles produced. The solution is stirred to no bubbles escaped from solution. The carboxyl group of aspirin reacts with sodium bicarbonate and the sodium aspirin forms. If some solids can not be dissolved during this operation, the solids are filtered out and the filtered cake was washed with a small amount of water. Concentrated hydrochloric acid 17.5ml and water 15ml are added to another 150ml beaker. The above filtrate is poured into this beaker in several times with stirring at the same time. A white solid, aspirin, precipitated (Note 5). The beaker is cooled with ice – bath fully to make aspirin precipitate completely. The precipitate is filtrated under reduced pressure and washed with a little cold water. Then the solid is pressed tight and dried. The crude product of aspirin is gained, mp. 135 ~ 136℃.

The above crude product of aspirin is put into a 25ml erlenmeyer flask. A little amount (less than 15ml) of hot ethyl acetate is added and two pieces of zeolite are also added. The solution is slowly heated to boil and the solid is just dissolved. Then the solution is cooled to room temperature, or cooled with ice – bath, aspirin is precipitated gradually (Note 6). After filtration, the pure aspirin is obtained. (Note 7)

3. Notes

Note 1: It may be heated with steam – bath, hot – plate, electrothermal pot or water – bath. If the heating medium used is water, it should be careful to prevent steam entering the flask, otherwise acetic anhydride and aspirin will be hydrolyzed.

Note 2: If no aspirin solid appears during cooling to room temperature, we may scrape inside the flask gently with glass rod, or put the flask into ice – bath, then the aspirin crystal will form.

Note 3: The water should only be added after the crystal formed fully. The adding of water is exothermal, the solution will become warm, hot and even boiling and the smoke of acetic acid will be given out. So the adding of water should be conducted carefully under ventilated condition.

Note 4: The beaker should be cooled with ice – bath to remove the producing heat. Since great amount of bubble will come out, thus the saturated sodium bicarbonate aqueous solution should be added in portion with stirring to prevent carbon dioxide foam overflow.

Note 5: If no solid appears, the pH of the solution should be tested. If the solution is not acidic, more hydrochloric acid should be added until the pH is about 2, and then the solid will come out.

Note 6: If no solid appears, the solution can be heated to evaporate a little amount of ethyl acetate.

Note 7: The purity test of aspirin: Two clean tubes are taken, a little salicylic acid and aspirin product are put into each respectively. Then ethanol 1ml is added into both tubes to dissolve the solid. Several drops of 10% solution of $FeCl_3$ are added into each tube. Since there is a hydroxyl group in salicylic acid, the solution in the tube containing salicylic acid will turn to red or purple. The color of the solution in the tube containing aspirin will be colorless, because the hydroxyl group of aspirin has been acetylated.

4. Questions　　What is the mechanism of the production of polymer? Are there any other byproducts besides the polymer?

【Characterization of Asprin】

Melting point: 136 ~ 140℃.

$^1H - NMR$: Conforms (Attached figure 4 – 1).

HRMS(ESI$^+$): 203.0031(M + Na$^+$)(Attached figure 4 – 2).

HPLC purity: 99.9%.

HPLC conditions:

Column: C18(4.6mm × 250mm, 5μm).

Flow rate: 1.0ml/min.

Injection volume: 10μl.

Detection wavelength: 303nm.

Mobile phase: Acetonitrile – tetrahydrofuran – glacial acetic acid – water(20 : 5 : 5 : 70).
Ultrasonic degassing before use.

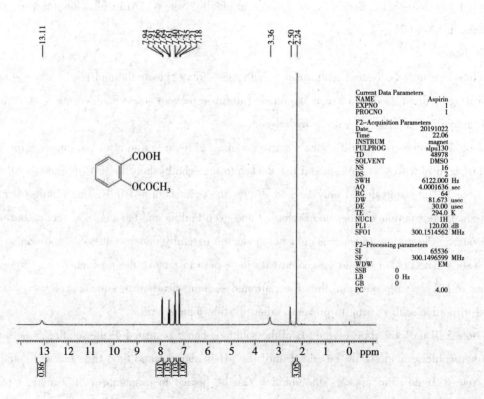

Attached figure 4 – 1　$^1H – NMR$ spectrum of aspirin(DMSO – d_6)

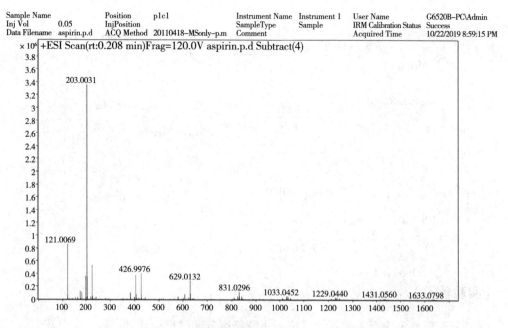

Sample Name　　　　　　Position　　p1c1　　　　　Instrument Name　Instrument 1　　User Name　　　　　G6520B-PC\Admin
Inj Vol　　0.05　　　　　　InjPosition　　　　　　　SampleType　　　Sample　　　　　IRM Calibration Status　Success
Data Filename　aspirin.p.d　ACQ Method　20110418-MSonly-p.m　Comment　　　　　　　　　　Acquired Time　　　10/22/2019 8:59:15 PM

×10⁶ +ESI Scan(rt:0.208 min)Frag=120.0V aspirin.p.d Subtract(4)

203.0031

121.0069

426.9976

629.0132

831.0296

1033.0452

1229.0440

1431.0560

1633.0798

Attached figure 4 – 2　　HRMS spectrum of aspirin（ESI⁺）

扫码"学一学"

实验五　贝诺酯的合成

【实验目的】

1. 了解拼合原理在药物化学中的应用，了解酯化反应在药物化学结构修饰中的应用。

2. 通过本实验，熟悉酯化反应的方法，掌握无水操作的技能。

3. 通过本实验，掌握反应中产生有害气体的吸收方法。

【实验原理】

贝诺酯（benorilate）的化学名为 2 – 乙酰氧基苯甲酸 4 – 乙酰氨基苯酯，［4 – acetamidophenyl 2 – acetoxybenzoate］，又称苯乐来。化学结构式为：

贝诺酯为白色结晶或结晶性粉末，mp. 177 ~ 181℃，在沸乙醇中易溶，在沸甲醇中溶解，在甲醇或乙醇中微溶，在水中不溶。

贝诺酯是由阿司匹林和乙酰氨基酚为原料合成制备的，将乙酰氨基酚的酚羟基和阿司匹林的羧酸基反应形成酯键。阿司匹林是芳香酸，反应性较低。反应中，先将阿司匹林在无水条件下与氯化亚砜、吡啶反应制得乙酰水杨酰氯（5 – 1）。再将反应活性较低的乙酰氨基酚的酚羟基与氢氧化钠反应形成酚钠盐（5 – 2）。然后，将（5 – 1）和（5 – 2）在室温下反应合成贝诺酯。

反应式（5-1）、（5-2）及贝诺酯合成示意

【实验预习】

1. 预习有机化学中有关酰氯化反应，由酰氯制备酯的反应原理。
2. 预习药物化学中有关酯化修饰在药物结构修饰中的作用和意义。
3. 预习减压蒸馏的原理和方法。
4. 预习无水操作反应及反应中产生有害气体的常用吸收方法。

【知识点】

仪器装置，投料过程，酰化反应，酯化反应，有害气体吸收，纯度检查。

【实验步骤】

1. 原料规格及配比　见表5-1。

表5-1　原料规格及配比表

原料名称	规格	用量	摩尔数	摩尔比
阿司匹林	药用	9g	0.05	1
氯化亚砜	CP，bp.78.8℃	5ml	0.05	1
吡啶	CP	1滴	0.005	0.1
对乙酰氨基酚	药用	8.6g	0.057	1.13
氢氧化钠	CP	3.3g	0.078	1.55
丙酮	AR，bp.56.5℃	6ml	0.081	1.63

　2. 实验操作　在装有回流冷凝器（上端附有氯化钙干燥管、排气导管通入氢氧化钠溶液）、温度计的150ml三颈瓶中（附注1），加入止爆剂、阿司匹林9g、氯化亚砜5ml（附注2），滴入吡啶1滴（附注3）（催化反应用），置油浴上缓缓加热，在50分钟左右升至75℃，维持70~75℃（附注4），搅拌至无气体逸出（2~3小时）。反应毕改成减压蒸馏装置用水泵减压，减压蒸除过量的氯化亚砜后（防止倒吸）（附注5），冷却至室

温，加入无水丙酮6ml（附注6），得含有乙酰水杨酰氯的丙酮溶液（5-1），混匀密封备用。

另取一个装有搅拌器、恒压滴液漏斗、温度计的150ml三颈瓶，加入对乙酰氨基酚8.6g，水50ml，搅拌下，于10~15℃，缓缓滴加氢氧化钠水溶液18ml（氢氧化钠3.3g加水至18ml），得到乙酰氨基酚钠水溶液（5-2）。将装有（5-2）水溶液的三颈瓶降温至8~12℃，慢慢滴加上述制得的乙酰水杨酰氯无水丙酮液（5-1）（约20分钟滴毕），调节反应液pH=9~10，于20~25℃搅拌1.5~2小时。反应毕，抽滤，用水洗至中性，烘干，得粗品。

将粗品放入100ml烧瓶中，加入95%乙醇（样品：95%乙醇=1:8），加热使样品恰好溶解，将溶液冷至室温，使样品析出，抽滤，得贝诺酯精品5~7g，mp.177~181℃，收率：44%。

3. 附注

（1）本反应是无水操作，所用仪器必须事先干燥，这是关系到本实验能否成功的关键。在酰氯化反应中，氯化亚砜作用后，放出氯化氢和二氧化硫气体，刺激性、腐蚀性较强，若不吸收，污染空气，损害健康，所以应用碱液吸收。

（2）为了便于搅拌，观察内温，使反应更趋完全，可适当增加氯化亚砜用量至6~7ml。

（3）吡啶仅起催化作用，不得过多，否则影响产品的质量和产量。

（4）在反应过程中，注意控制反应温度在70~75℃为佳，不宜超过80℃。反应温度太低，不利于反应进行，温度太高氯化亚砜易挥发。

（5）在减压蒸除氯化亚砜时应注意观察，防止水泵压力变化引起水倒吸。若发现水倒吸进接受瓶，应立即将接受瓶取下，放入水槽中用大量水冲洗稀释。切勿将接受瓶密塞。因为氯化亚砜见水后分解放出大量氯化氢气体。

$$SOCl_2 + 2H_2O \longrightarrow 2HCl + SO_2$$

（6）分析纯丙酮加入炒过的无水硫酸钠干燥后即可。

4. 思考题

（1）由羧酸制备酰氯常用哪些方法？

（2）在由羧酸和氯化亚砜反应制备酰氯时，为什么要加少量的吡啶？吡啶量若加多了会发生什么后果，为什么？

（3）什么叫拼合原理？在药物化学中有什么意义？

【贝诺酯的结构表征】

熔点：177~181℃。

^{1}H-NMR：结构正确（附图5-1~5-3）。

HRMS（ESI$^+$）：314.0987（M+H$^+$）（附图5-4）。

HPLC纯度：99.9%

HPLC测试的色谱条件：

色谱柱：十八烷基硅烷键合硅胶（150mm×4.6mm，5μm）。

流速：1.0ml/min。

进样量：10μl。

检测波长：245nm。

柱温：35℃。

流动相：以水（用磷酸调节 pH 至 3.5）–甲醇（44∶56）为流动相。使用前需超声脱气。

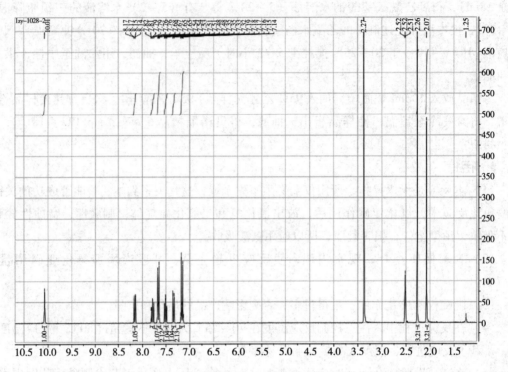

附图 5 – 1　贝诺酯的¹H – NMR 谱图（DMSO – d₆）

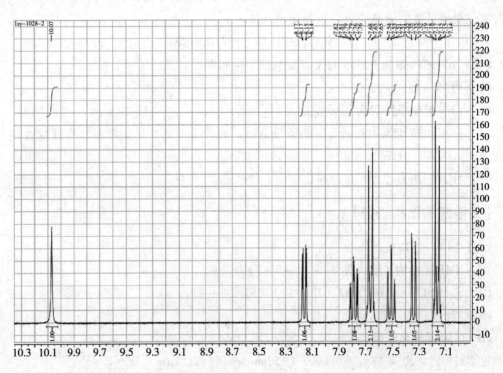

附图 5 – 2　贝诺酯的¹H – NMR（局部）谱图（DMSO – d₆）

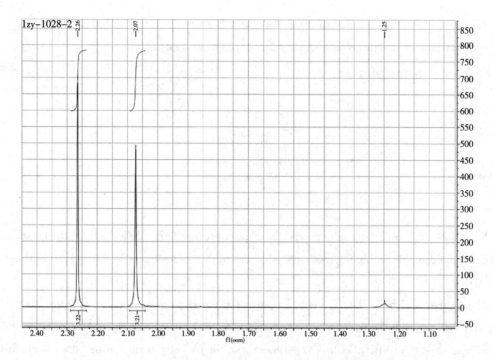

附图 5-3　贝诺酯的 ^{1}H-NMR（局部）谱图（DMSO-d$_6$）

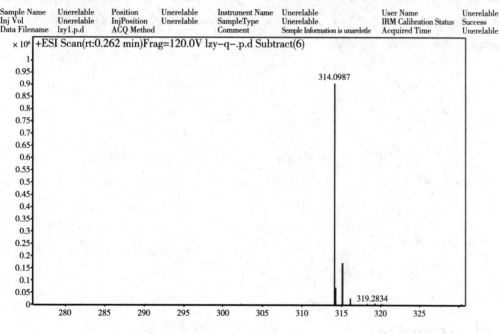

附图 5-4　贝诺酯的 HRMS 谱图（ESI$^+$）

Experiment 5　　Synthesis of Benorilate

Experimental aim

1. Learn the application of twin-drug in the medicinal chemistry and the application of esterification in structure modification.

扫码"学一学"

2. Train the operation of esterification and the anhydrous operation technique.

3. Learn how to absorb poisonous gas released from the reaction.

Experimental principles

Benorilate

4 – acetamidophenyl 2 – acetoxybenzoate

Benorilate is a white crystal or crystalline powder, mp. 177 ~ 181℃. It is freely soluble in boiling ethanol, soluble in boiling methanol, slightly soluble in methanol or ethanol, and insoluble in water.

The synthesis of benorilate is started from aspirin and paracetamol. The phenol group of the paracetamol reacts with the carbonyl group of aspirin to form an ester product. Aspirin is an aromatic acid which has low reactivity. In this experiment, aspirin is firstly treated with thionyl chloride and pyridine to prepare the corresponding acetyl salicylic chloride (5 – 1) in anhydrous condition. Considering the similar low reactivity of phenol group of the paracetamol, paracetamol is turned to its sodium salt(5 – 2) in sodium hydroxide solution. Then(5 – 1) reacts with(5 – 2) in room temperature to form benorilate.

Pre – lab preparation

1. Review the preparation principle of esters from acid chlorides in organic chemistry.

2. Summary the role and significance of esterification modification in drug structure modification in medicinal chemistry.

3. Review the process and operation of vacuum distillation.

4. Review the operation of anhydrous reaction and the common absorption apparatus of harmful gases generated in the reaction.

Knowledge point

Set – up of reaction apparatus, adding procedures of chemical reagents, acylation reaction, esterification reaction, harmful gas absorption, purity check.

Experiment procedures

1. Materials(Table 5 – 1)

Table 5 – 1　Specification and ratio of raw materials

Materials	Specifications	Amount	Mol	Mol ratio
Aspirin	Medicinal grade	9g	0.05	1
Thionyl chloride	CP, bp. 78.8℃	5ml	0.05	1
Pyridine	CP	1drop	0.005	0.1
Paracetamol	Medicinal grade	8.6g	0.057	1.13
Sodium hydroxide	CP	3.3g	0.078	1.55
Anhydrous acetone	AR, bp. 56.5℃	6ml	0.081	1.63

2. Procedures　To a 150ml three – necked flask equipped with arefluxing condenser and a thermometer(Note 1), aspirin 9g, thionyl chloride 5ml(Note 2) and some pieces of zeolite are added, and then a drop of pyridine is also added(Note 3). The reaction solution is heated slowly on the oil – bath. The temperature will rise to 70 ~ 75℃ (Note 4) in about 50 minutes and such temperature will be maintained until no gas is released(about 2 ~ 3h). The equipped flask was changed from refluxing to vacuum distillation. The excess thionyl chloride and other gases produced in the reaction are distilled by exhaustion with a water pump(Note 5). After the reaction mixture is cooled to the room temperature, anhydrous acetone 6ml(Note 6) is added into the flask, then the flask containing acetyl salicylic chloride(5 – 1) for the forward step is sealed.

To another 150ml four – necked flask equipped with a stirring, a refluxing condenser, a thermometer and a dropping funnel, paracetamol 8.6g and water 50ml are added. A solution of sodium hydroxide 3.3g in water 18ml is added into the flask slowly by the dropping funnel at 10 ~ 15℃ with stirring. After the addition of sodium hydroxide aqueous solution, a solution of(5 – 2) is formed. Then, the flask of(5 – 2) solution is cooled to 8 ~ 12℃ and the above anhydrous acetone solution of the acetyl salicylic chloride (5 – 1) is slowly added to the mixture through another dropping funnel at 8 ~ 12℃ (about 20 minutes). After dropping, the pH of the reaction mixture is adjusted to 9 ~ 10 and the reaction mixture is stirred between 20 to 25℃ for another 1.5 ~ 2.0 hours. The reaction mixture is filtrated, and the filtering cake is washed with water until the pH value of the filtrate reaches about 7. After dried under infrared light, the crude product of benorilate is obtained.

The crude product is put into a 100ml flask, and 95% ethanol is also added in several portions. The volume of the alcohol is determined by the quantity of the product, about 95% ethanol 8ml for product 1g. The crude product will be just completely dissolved in the boiling ethanol. After the product is dissolved, the heating bath is removed and the flask is cooled to room temperature. Then the flask is cooled in the ice bath until benorilate is precipitated completely. The pure benorilate (about 5 ~ 7g, mp. 177 ~ 181℃) is obtained after filtration and dried under the infrared lamp.

3. Notes

Note 1: Because thionyl chloride and the produced acetyl salicylic chloride are sensitive to moisture, the reaction should be carried out under anhydrous condition. All the equipments and materials should be dried beforehand and a calcium chloride drying tube should be installed on the top of the refluxing condenser. Since a large amount of gaseous hydrogen chloride and sulfur dioxide will generate in the reaction, an additional apparatus is required to absorb the acidic gas by sodium hydroxide aqueous solution through guiding tube.

Note 2: Increasing the amount of thionyl chloride to 6 ~ 7ml can make stirring easier and the reaction more complete.

Note 3: Pyridine is only used as catalyst. If it is used too much, the quality and yield of the product will be influenced.

Note 4: The reaction temperature should be kept at 70 ~ 75℃ and shouldn't exceed 80℃. Too high temperature will lead to the volatilization of thionyl chloride and the formation of polymer, where as too low temperature is unfavorable for the reaction.

Note 5: Any changes of exhaustion pressure will cause water flowing back to distillation system. Carefully observe to prevent water flowing back. If water flows back to the receiving flask of distillation system, the flask should be taken away immediately and rinsed with large amount of water. It is very dangerous to stopper the flask tightly, because thionyl chloride will be decomposed to produce large amount of gaseous hydrogen chloride and sulfur dioxide.

$$SOCl_2 + 2H_2O \longrightarrow 2HCl + SO_2$$

Note 6: Anhydrous acetone could be prepared by adding new parched anhydrous sodium sulfate to analytical pure acetone.

4. Questions

(1) What are the preparation methods of carboxylic chloride from carboxylic acid?

(2) Why should some pyridine be added in the preparation of acetyl salicylic chloride from salicylic acid and thionly chloride? What would happen if the pyridine is added more excess?

(3) What is the principle of Twin – drug? Please give some examples in drug research.

【Characterization of Benorilate】

Melting point: 177 ~ 181℃.
^{1}H – NMR: Conformed(Attached figure 5 – 1 ~ 5 – 3).
HRMS(ESI$^+$):314.0987(M + H$^+$)(Attached figure 5 – 4).
HPLC purity: 99.9%.

HPLC conditions:
Column: C18(150mm × 4.6mm,5μm).
Flow rate: 1.0ml/min.
Injection volume: 10μl.
Detection wavelength: 245nm.
Column temperature: 35℃.
Mobile phase: Using water(regulating pH value with phosphoric acid to 3.5) – methanol(44:

56）as mobile phase. Ultrasonic degassing before use.

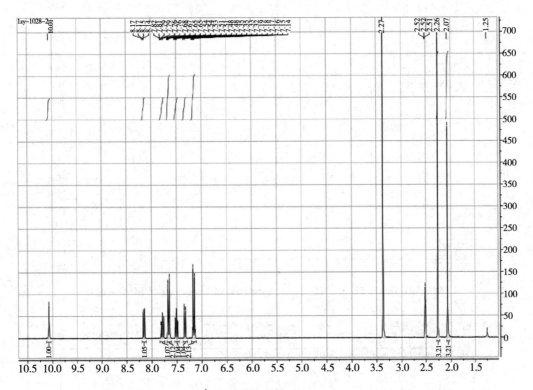

Attached figure 5 – 1　^{1}H – NMR spectrum of benorilate(DMSO – d$_6$)

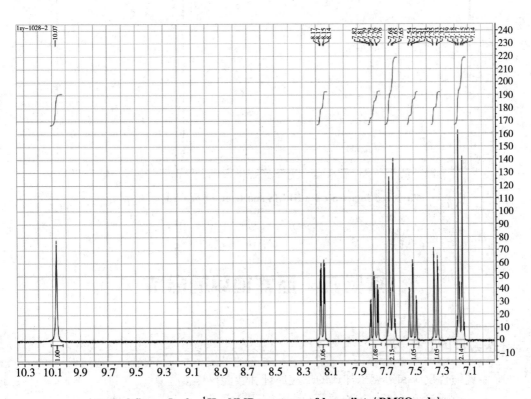

Attached figure 5 – 2　^{1}H – NMR spectrum of benorilate(DMSO – d$_6$)

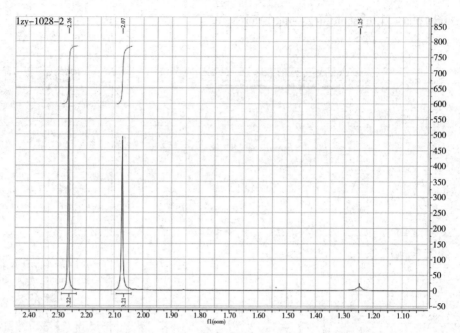

Attached figure 5 – 3   ¹H – NMR spectrum of benorilate(DMSO – d₆)

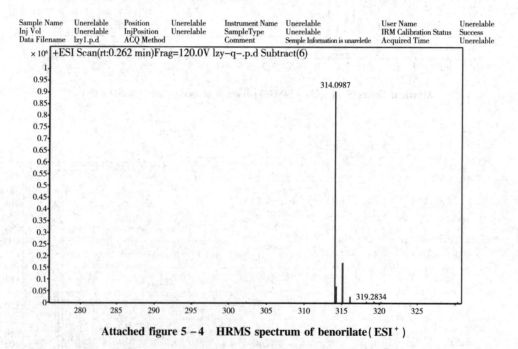

Attached figure 5 – 4   HRMS spectrum of benorilate(ESI⁺)

实验六   尼群地平的合成

【实验目的】

1. 掌握缩合反应和迈克尔加成的反应原理和实验操作。

2. 分析尼群地平中杂质的主要来源。

3. 掌握氮气保护在合成反应中的作用。

【实验原理】

尼群地平（nitrendipine）的化学名为 2，6 - 二甲基 - 4 - （3 - 硝基苯基） - 1，4 - 二氢 - 3，5 - 吡啶二甲酸甲乙酯，[3 - ethyl 5 - methyl 2，6 - dimethyl - 4 - （3 - nitrophenyl） - 1，4 - dihydropyridine - 3，5 - dicarboxylate]。化学结构式为：

尼群地平为黄色结晶粉末，熔点：157 ~ 161℃。遇光易变质。在丙酮或三氯甲烷中易溶，在甲醇或乙醇中略溶，在水中几乎不溶。

尼群地平的合成是以 3 - 硝基苯甲醛（6 - 1）和乙酰乙酸乙酯为起始原料。在酸催化下，3 - 硝基苯甲醛和乙酰乙酸乙酯缩合得 2 - （3 - 硝基苄亚基）乙酰乙酸乙酯（6 - 2）。然后，（6 - 2）和 3 - 氨基丁烯酸甲酯在无水乙醇加热至回流，得尼群地平。

二氢吡啶类化合物（如，1，4 - 二氢吡啶类钙通道阻滞剂）中的二氢吡啶环对光和热比较敏感，在环合过程中易氧化为吡啶化合物，因此反应时应尽量避光，且最好在氮气流保护下反应。另外，当 3，5 位的酯基不同时，还会发生不同程度的酯交换反应，生成少量双甲酯和双乙酯副产物。

【实验预习】

1. 二氢吡啶环的合成主要有哪些方法？
2. 缩合反应和迈克尔加成的反应原理是什么？
3. 简述尼群地平的理化性质。

【知识点】

仪器装置，投料过程，缩合反应，迈克尔加成反应，氮气保护。

【实验步骤】

（一）3-硝基亚苄基乙酰乙酸乙酯的制备

1. 原料规格及配比　见表6-1。

表6-1　原料规格及配比表

原料名称	规格	用量	摩尔数	摩尔比
3-硝基苯甲醛（6-1）	CP	7.6g	0.05	1
乙酰乙酸乙酯	CP	9.8g	0.075	1.5
乙酸酐	CP	5.1g	0.05	1
浓硫酸	CP	1.2g	0.012	0.24
95%乙醇	CP	10ml		

2. 实验操作　在装有搅拌器、温度计和恒压滴液漏斗的50ml三颈瓶（附注1）中，依次加入乙酰乙酸乙酯和乙酸酐，用冰浴冷却至0℃（附注2），搅拌下缓慢滴加浓硫酸，10分钟后，分5~10次加入3-硝基苯甲醛（附注3），期间保持温度不超过5℃，滴加完毕后，自然升温至室温（附注4），室温保温搅拌1小时。加入95%乙醇10ml，搅拌下于10分钟内冷却至0~5℃，在该温度下保温搅拌0.5小时，抽滤，所得固体用冷95%乙醇洗涤2次（附注5），再用冷水洗涤至pH 6，自然晾干，得类白色固体（6-2），mp. 107~109℃，称重，计算收率。

3. 附注

（1）水会影响反应的进行，所有仪器应干燥。

（2）如用冰盐浴，冷却效果会更好。

（3）反应温度如能控制在5℃以下，加入3-硝基苯甲醛的速度可以适当加快。

（4）反应液变为透明并逐渐变得黏稠。

（5）每次洗涤时，冷95%乙醇的用量在3ml左右，太多的话会溶解部分产品，影响收率；但也不能太少，太少的话会影响产品的色泽。

4. 思考题

（1）乙酸酐在本反应所起的主要作用是什么？能否用其他试剂代替？

（2）浓硫酸在本反应起什么作用？能否用其他酸代替？

（二）尼群地平的制备

1. 原料规格及配比　见表6-2。

表6-2　原料规格及配比表

原料名称	规格	用量	摩尔数	摩尔比
3-硝基亚苄基乙酰乙酸乙酯（6-2）	自制	5.3g	0.02	1
β-氨基巴豆酸甲酯	CP	2.8g	0.024	1.2

续表

原料名称	规格	用量	摩尔数	摩尔比
无水乙醇	CP	18ml		
浓盐酸	CP	0.4g		
自来水		10ml		

2. 实验操作　在装有回流冷凝管和温度计的50ml三颈瓶（附注1）中，依次加入3-硝基亚苄基乙酰乙酸乙酯（6-2）、β-氨基巴豆酸甲酯（附注2）和无水乙醇18ml，加入少量人工沸石，加热回流（附注3）1小时，加入浓盐酸0.4ml，继续回流反应0.5小时，稍冷，滴加自来水10ml，慢慢冷却（附注4）析晶，并于0~5℃放置2小时（附注5），抽滤，晶体用冰50%乙醇洗涤3~5次（附注6），真空干燥，得淡黄色晶体，mp.157~159℃，称重，计算收率。

3. 附注

（1）水会影响反应的进行，影响产品的收率和质量，故所有仪器使用前应干燥。

（2）β-氨基巴豆酸甲酯的制备：将乙酰乙酸甲酯100ml（0.93mol），无水乙醇20ml加入250ml四颈瓶中，冰盐浴冷却至0℃，通干燥氨气至饱和，约4小时通毕，冷冻过夜，抽滤，晶体用无水甲醇重结晶得白色结晶85~89g，mp.82~83℃。

（3）通氮气保护，产品质量更好。

（4）冷却速度越慢，析出的产品质量越好。

（5）如在冰箱中放置过夜，收率会有所提高。

（6）50%乙醇最好预先冷却至-15℃左右，否则会溶解部分产品，影响收率。

4. 思考题

（1）浓盐酸在本反应起什么作用？能否用其他酸代替??

（2）如用无水甲醇为反应溶剂，对反应结果是否有影响？

【尼群地平的结构表征】

熔点：157.8~161.2℃。

^{1}H-NMR：结构正确（附图6-1）。

HRMS（ESI$^+$）：383.0（M+Na$^+$）（附图6-2）。

HPLC纯度：99.9%。

HPLC测试的色谱条件：

色谱柱：Hypersil C18（4.6mm×250mm，5μm）。

流速：1.0ml/min。

进样量：10μl。

检测波长：227nm。

柱温：室温。

流动相：甲醇-水（体积比为70∶30）。使用前需超声脱气。

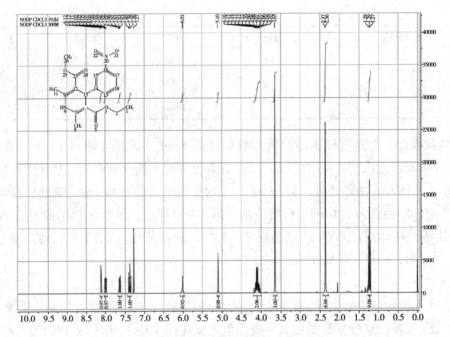

附图 6 - 1　尼群地平的 ^{1}H - NMR 谱图（CDCl$_3$）

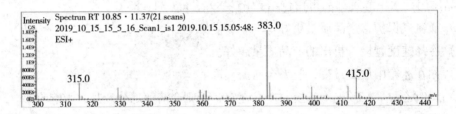

附图 6 - 2　尼群地平的 HRMS 谱图（ESI$^+$）

Experiment 6　Synthesis of Nitrendipine

Experimental aim

1. Learn the principles and the operations of condensation reaction and Michael Addition.

2. Analyze the main source of the impurities in nitrendipine.

3. Learn the application of nitrogen gas protection in organic synthesis.

Experimental principles

Nitrendipine

3 - ethyl 5 - methyl 2,6 - dimethyl - 4 - (3 - nitrophenyl) - 1,

4 - dihydropyridine - 3,5 - dicarboxylate

Nitrendipine is a yellow crystalline powder with mp. 156 ~ 160℃. It is easy deteriorated in light. It is freely soluble in acetone or chloroform, sparingly soluble in methanol or ethanol, practically insoluble in water.

Synthesis ofnitrendipine was from nitrobenzaldehyde(6 - 1) and ethyl acetoacetate as starting materials. Ethyl 2 - (3 - nitrobenzylidene)acetoacetate(6 - 2) was obtained by condensation of 3 - nitrobenzaldehyde and ethyl acetoacetate under the catalysis of acid. Then, (6 - 2) and 3 - aminobutenoic acid methyl ester are heated and refluxed in anhydrous ethanol and nitrendipine is obtained.

The dihydropyridine ring in 1, 4 - dihydropyridine derivatives (such as 1, 4 - dihydropyridine calcium channel blockers) is sensitive to light and heat. It tends to be oxidized to pyridine in the process of cyclization. So the reaction should be away from light and under the protection of nitrogen gas. In addition, when 3 - and 5 - ester group are different from each other, ester exchange reaction will happen and produce some by - product of dimethylester and diethylester.

Pre – lab preparation

1. Summary and compare the synthesis pathway of dihydropyridine.

2. Learn the principle of Michael Addition and condensation reaction in this experiment.

3. Learn the main physico – chemical properties of nitrendipine.

Knowledge point

Set – up of reaction apparatus, adding procedures of chemical reagents, condensation reaction, Michael Addition, nitrogen protection.

Experimental procedures

I. Synthesis of ethyl 3 – nitrobenzylidene acetoacetate(6 – 2)

1. Materials(Table 6 – 1)

Table 6 – 1   Specification and ratio of raw materials

Materials	Specifications	Amount	Mol	Mol ratio
3 – nitrobenzaldehyde(6 – 1)	CP	7.6g	0.05	1
Ethyl acetoacetate	CP	9.8g	0.075	1.5
Acetic anhydride	CP	5.1g	0.05	1
Concentrated sulfuric acid	CP	1.2g	0.012	0.24
95% ethanol	CP	10ml		

2. Procedures   To a 50ml three – necked flask(Note 1)equipped with a stirrer, a thermometer and a dropping funnel, ethyl acetoacetate and acetic anhydride are added. After the mixture is cooled to 0℃ with an ice bath(Note 2), concentrated sulfuric acid is added dropwise by dropping funnel under stirring. 10 min later, 3 – nitrobenzaldehyde is added in 5 ~ 10 batches(Note 3). The reaction temperature should be kept below 5℃ during addition of 3 – nitrobenzaldehyde. After completing addition of 3 – nitrobenzaldehyde, the reaction temperature should be raised to room temperature (Note 4)and the reaction mixture is stirred at room temperature for another 1h. Then, 95% ethanol 10ml is added, and the reaction mixture is cooled to 0 ~ 5℃ in 10 min and maintained for 0.5h. The reaction mixture is filtered, and the filter cake is washed two times with ice – cold 95% ethanol (Note 5), and then washed with ice – cold water to pH 6. The off – white solid(6 – 2)can be obtained after dried over air flow, mp. 107 ~ 109℃, weigh and calculate yield.

3. Notes

Note 1: All instruments should be dried before use, for the presence of water would bring a disadvantageous effect on reaction.

Note 2: The cooling effect with ice – salt bath would be better than that of ice bath.

Note 3: If the reaction temperature is well controlled below 5℃, the addition of 3 – nitrobenzaldehyde can be in a moderately quick rate.

Note 4: The reaction mixture become transparent and then viscous gradually.

Note 5: The volume of ice – cold 95% ethanol is about 3ml each time. Too much will dissolve part of product to affect the yield, and too little will influence the colour and lustre of product.

4. Questions

(1)What is the main role of acetic anhydride in this reaction? Can it be replaced by other reagent?

(2)What is the role of concentrated sulfuric acid in the reaction? Can it be replaced by other acid?

Ⅱ. Preparation of Nitrendipine

1. Materials(Table 6 – 2)

Table 6 – 2 Specification and ratio of raw materials

Materials	Specifications	Amount	Mol	Mol ratio
3 – nitrobenzylidene acetoacetate(6 – 2)	Self – prepared	5.3g	0.02	1
Methyl 3 – aminocrotonate	CP	2.8g	0.024	1.2
Anhydrousethanol	CP	18ml		
Concentrated hydrochloric acid	CP	0.4ml		
Water		10ml		

2. Procedures

To a 50ml three – necked flask(Note 1) equipped with a condenser and a thermometer,3 – nitrobenzylidene acetoacetate(6 – 2), methyl 3 – aminocrotonate(Note 2) and anhydrous ethanol 18ml are added in turn. The reaction mixture is stirred with magnetic stirring and refluxed for 1h(Note 3). Concentrated hydrochloric acid 0.4ml is added, and the mixture is refluxed for another 0.5h. Water 10ml is added dropwise, and the mixture is cooled down to room temperature slowly(Note 4), and then kept at $0 \sim 5\,^{\circ}\!C$ for 2h(Note 5). The precipitate is collected by suction and washed three to five times with ice – cold 50% ethanol(Note 6). Dried in vacuo to give light – yellow crystal,mp. $157 \sim 159\,^{\circ}\!C$,weigh and calculate yield.

3. Notes

Note 1:All instruments should be dried before use, for the presence of water would bring a disadvantageous effect on yield and quality of nitrendipine.

Note 2:Preparation of methyl 3 – aminocrotonate:To a 250ml four – necked flask equipped with a stirrer, a thermometer and a drying tube containing drying agent, methyl acetoacetate 100ml (0.93mol)and anhydrous ethanol 20ml are added. The reaction mixture is cooled below $0\,^{\circ}\!C$ with ice – salt bath, and then is saturated with gaseous ammonia which needs about 4h. The resultant mixture is kept between $0\,^{\circ}\!C$ and $5\,^{\circ}\!C$ overnight. The crude crystal is collected by suction and recrystallized from anhydrous methanol to give $85 \sim 89g$ of methyl 3 – aminocrotonate as a white crystal. mp. $82 \sim 83\,^{\circ}\!C$.

Note 3:The quality of product will be better under the protection of nitrogen gas.

Note 4:The more slowly the solution cools down, the better the quality of product is.

Note 5:The yield can be improved if the reaction mixture is kept in refrigeratory over night.

Note 6:50% ethanol should be precooled to $-15\,^{\circ}\!C$, or it may dissolve some product and decrease the yield.

4. Questions

(1)What is the role of concentrated hydrochloric acid in the reaction? Can it be replaced by other acid?

(2)Does it influence reaction result if we use anhydrous methanol as the reaction solvent?

【Characterization of Nitrendipine】

Melting point:157.8 ~ 161.2℃.

^{1}H – NMR：Conforms（Attached figure 6 – 1）.

HRMS（ESI$^+$）：380.0（M + Na$^+$）（Attached figure 6 – 2）.

HPLC purity：99.9%.

HPLC conditions：

Column：Hypersil C18（4.6mm × 250mm,5μm）.

Flow rate：1.0ml/min.

Injection volume：10μl.

Detection wavelength：227nm.

Column temperature：Room temperatur.

Mobile phase：MeOH – H$_2$O（70∶30）.

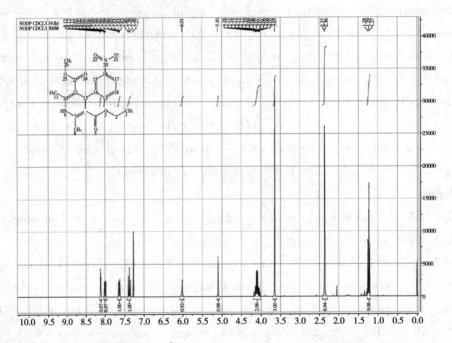

Attached figure 6 – 1 ^{1}H – NMR spectrum of nitrendipine（CDCl$_3$）

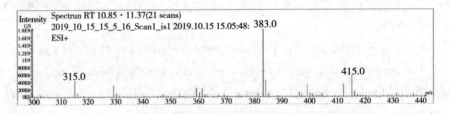

Attached figure 6 – 2   HRMS spectrum of nitrendipine（ESI$^+$）

实验七   依达拉奉的合成

【实验目的】

1. 熟悉吡唑环的合成原理。

2. 了解无水苯肼的性质和使用注意事项。

【实验原理】

依达拉奉（edaravone）的化学名为3 - 甲基 - 1 - 苯基 - 2 - 吡唑啉 - 5 - 酮，[3 - methyl - 1 - phenyl - 2 - pyrazolin - 5 - one]。化学结构式为：

$$\text{（结构式）}$$

依达拉奉是一种白色或类白色结晶性粉末，mp. 128 ~ 130℃。溶于甲醇和乙醇，几乎不溶于水。

依达拉奉是一种自由基清除剂，其良好的脑保护作用已得到国内外临床研究的证实，临床上用于改善急性脑梗塞所致的神经症状、日常生活活动能力和功能障碍。

依达拉奉的合成是由苯肼和乙酰乙酸乙酯在乙醇中加热环合得到。

$$\text{（反应式）} \quad (1)\ CH_3COCH_2COOC_2H_5/C_2H_5OH \quad (2)\ conc.\ HCl \quad (3)\ 10\%NaOH \longrightarrow \text{依达拉奉}$$

游离的苯肼不稳定，在空气中易发生潮解和氧化反应，需密闭避光贮存，使用时应迅速转移到真空滴液漏斗中，在滴加过程中通氮气保护。

【实验预习】

1. 总结依达拉奉的合成路线，并比较本实验中所采用的路线与其他路线的优缺点。
2. 简述依达拉奉的合成原理。

【知识点】

仪器装置，投料过程，酸碱调节，纯度检测，TLC 检测。

【实验步骤】

1. 原料规格及配比 见表7 - 1。

表7 - 1 原料规格及配比表

原料名称	规格	用量	摩尔数	摩尔比
苯肼	CP	10.8g	0.1	1
乙酰乙酸乙酯	CP	13.0g	0.1	1
70% 乙醇	自制	5ml		
无水乙醇	CP	3ml		
浓盐酸	AR	1ml		
10% NaOH	自制	适量		

2. 实验操作　在装有搅拌器、温度计和 25ml 恒压滴液漏斗的 100ml 三颈瓶中，加入乙酰乙酸乙酯 13g（0.1mol）和 70% 乙醇 5ml。搅拌下，水浴加热至 45℃，滴加苯肼 10.8g（附注 1）和无水乙醇 3ml 组成的溶液，约 30 分钟滴毕，在 45℃ 保温搅拌 20 分钟。冷却至 20℃，滴加浓盐酸 1ml（附注 2），继续在 45℃ 保温反应 2 小时后，滴加 10% NaOH 至 pH 7（附注 3），加水 20ml，室温搅拌 1 小时，抽滤，晶体用冷无水乙醇洗涤二次（附注 4），干燥，得浅黄色结晶 13g 左右。

上述粗品用乙酸乙酯/无水乙醇（2∶1，30ml）重结晶（附注 5），得白色晶体 8～10g，mp. 128～130℃。

3. 附注

（1）游离的苯肼不稳定，接触空气冒烟并很快变质，操作应快速，在滴加过程中通氮气保护。

（2）浓盐酸 1ml 可用滴管直接滴加。

（3）一般在 pH 3～4 时就有晶体析出，应继续调节至 pH 7，尽量使用机械搅拌。

（4）每次用冷乙醇 10ml。

（5）重结晶时应加活性炭脱色，如一次重结晶所得产品颜色较深，可再重结晶一次，即可得到白色晶体。

4. 思考题

（1）苯肼在空气中不稳定的原因是什么？

（2）浓盐酸在本反应中起到什么作用？

【依达拉奉的结构表征】

熔点：128～130℃。

^{1}H-NMR：结构正确（附图 7-1）。

HRMS（ESI$^+$）：175.0863（M + H$^+$）（附图 7-2）。

HPLC 纯度：99.5%。

HPLC 测试的色谱条件：

色谱柱：SHISEIDO SPOI AR C18。

流速：1.0ml/min。

进样量：20μg。

检测波长：195mm。

柱温：25℃。

流动相：乙腈-磷酸盐缓冲液（5∶95）。使用前需超声脱气。

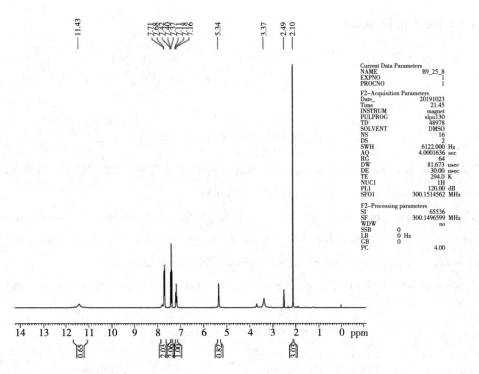

附图 7 – 1　依达拉奉的 ^{1}H – NMR 谱图（DMSO – d$_6$）

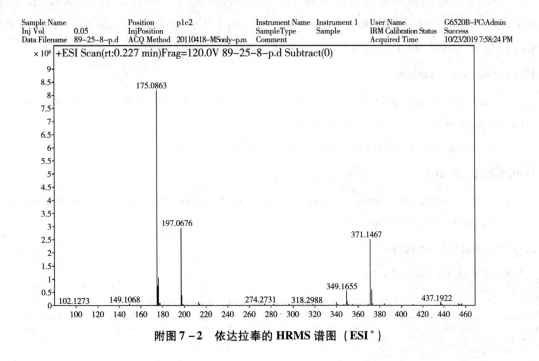

附图 7 – 2　依达拉奉的 HRMS 谱图（ESI$^+$）

Experiment 7　Synthesis of Edaravone

Experimental aim

1. Learn the synthetic principle of pyrazole ring.

2. Review the properties of phenylhydrazine and the precautions in use.

Experimental principles

O

Edaravone

$3 - methyl - 1 - phenyl - 2 - pyrazolin - 5 - one$

Edaravone is a white or off – white crystalline powder with mp. 128 ~ 130℃. It is soluble in methanol and ethanol and practically insoluble in water.

Edaravone is a free radical scavenger, and its good brain protection has been confirmed by clinical research at home and abroad. It is used to improve the neurological symptoms, activities of daily life and dysfunction caused by acute cerebral infarction in clinical.

Edaravone was synthesized by cyclization of phenylhydrazine and ethyl acetoacetate in ethanol.

$-NHNH_2$ $\xrightarrow[\substack{(2) \text{ conc. HCl} \\ (3) \ 10\%NaOH}]{(1) \ CH_3COCH_2COOC_2H_5/C_2H_5OH}$ Edaravone

Phenylhydrazine is unstable and prone to deliquescence and oxidation in the air. It needs to be stored in a closed place away from light. When it is used, it should be quickly transferred to the vacuum drop funnel and protected by nitrogen during the dropping process.

Pre – lab preparation

1. Summary the synthetic routes of edaravone and compare the advantages and disadvantages of the route used in this experiment with others.

2. Give a briefly describe the synthesis principle of edaravone.

Knowledge point

Set – up of reaction apparatus, adding procedures of chemical reagents, acid – base adjustment, purity detection, TLC detection.

Experiment procedures

1. Materials(Table 7 – 1)

Table 7 – 1 Specification and ratio of raw materials

Materials	Specifications	Amount	Mol	Mol ratio
Phenylhydrazine	CP	10. 8g	0. 1	1
Ethyl acetoacetate	CP	13. 0g	0. 1	1
Ethanol(70%)		5ml		
Absoluteethanol	CP	3ml		
Concentrated hydrochloric acid	AR	1ml		
Sodium hydroxide(10%)		Appropriate		

2. Procedures To a 100ml three – necked flask equipped with a stirrer, a thermometer and a 25ml dropping funnel, ethyl acetoacetate 13g and 70% ethanol 5ml are added in turn. The mixture is stirred and heated to about 45℃ by a water bath, and a solution of phenylhydrazine 10.8g(Note 1)in ethanol 3ml is added dropwise. The addition maintains about 30min, and the reaction mixture is stirred for another 20min at 45℃. The mixture is cooled to 20℃, concentrated hydrochloric acid 1ml is added(Note 2). The reaction mixture is stirred at 45℃ for 2h, and then 10% NaOH solution is added until the pH value reaches 7(Note 3). To the mixture, water 20ml is added, and stirring is maintained at room temperature for 1h, the resultant crystal is collected by suction and washed two times with ice–cold anhydrous ethanol(Note 4). Dried in vacuo to give about 13g of light–yellow crystal.

The crystalobtained is recrystallized with ethyl acetate/ethanol(2∶1,30ml)(Note 5), and 8g to 10g of edaravone as a white crystal can be obtained with mp. 128~130℃.

3. Notes

Note 1:Phenylhydrazine is not stable, and tends to be deliquated and oxidized in the air. So it should be stored away from air and light. It should transferred to dropping funnel quickly when using. Moreover, the addition should be under the protection of nitrogen gas.

Note 2:Concentrated hydrochloric acid 1ml could be added in one time with burette.

Note 3:There are crystals formed at pH 3~4, but it is necessary to adjust the pH of reaction mixture to 7 and stir with a mechanical stir.

Note 4:The volume of ice–cold ethanol is about 10ml each time.

Note 5:It is necessary that the solution should be decolorized with activated carbon. If the color of products is pale–yellow, recrystallization once again is necessary and white crystal can be obtained.

4. Questions

(1)Why is phenylhydrazine sensitive in the air?

(2)What is the role of concentrated hydrochloric acid in this reaction?

【Characterization of Edaravone】

Melting point:128~130℃.

^{1}H–NMR(300 MHz, DMSO–d$_6$):Conforms(Attached figure 7–1).

HRMS(ESI$^+$):175.0863(M + H$^+$)(Attached figure 7–2).

HPLC purity:99.5%.

HPLC conditions:

Column:SHISEIDO SPOI AR C18.

Flow rate:1.0ml/min.

Injection volume:20μg.

Detection wavelength:195mm.

Column temperature:25℃.

Mobile phase:Acetonitrile–phosphate buffer(5∶95).

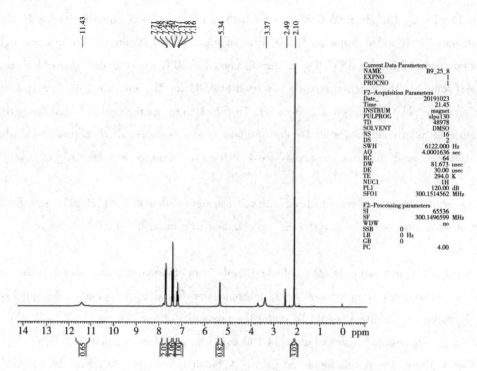

Attached figure 7 – 1 ^{1}H – NMR spectrum of edaravone(DMSO – d$_6$)

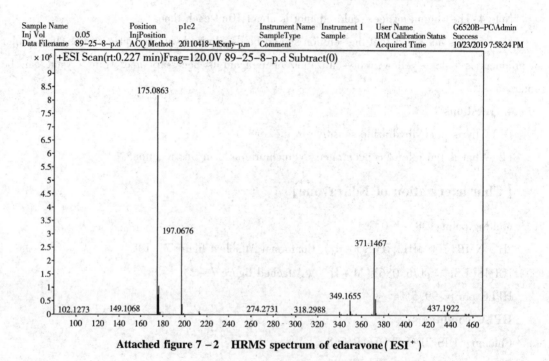

Attached figure 7 – 2   HRMS spectrum of edaravone(ESI$^+$)

实验八   美沙拉嗪的合成

【实验目的】

1. 通过本实验，掌握硝化反应的原理和实验操作。

2. 熟悉硝基还原的一般方法。

3. 熟悉美沙拉嗪的理化性质。

4. 了解保险粉的成分和用途。

【实验原理】

美沙拉嗪（mesalazine）的化学名为 5 - 氨基 - 2 - 羟基苯甲酸，[5 - amino - 2 - hydroxybenzoic acid]，别名：马沙拉嗪，5 - 氨基水杨酸（5 - amino salicylic acid），mp. 279 ~ 281℃。白色至粉红色结晶，熔点约 280℃（分解）。溶于盐酸，略溶于热水，微溶于冷水或乙醇。化学结构式如下：

美沙拉嗪的合成方法有多种，其中一种为水杨酸硝化还原法，反应式如下：

【实验预习】

1. 预习有机化学中的硝化反应，以及其反应机制。

2. 预习药物化学中有关硝基还原反应的药物合成路线。

3. 预习美沙拉嗪的理化性质。

【知识点】

仪器装置，投料过程，硝化反应，硝基还原反应，纯度检查。

【实验步骤】

（一）5 - 硝基水杨酸的制备

1. 原料规格及配比　如表 8 - 1。

表 8 - 1　原料规格及配比表

原料名称	规格	用量	摩尔数	摩尔比
水杨酸（8 - 1）	药用	13.8g	0.1	1
硝酸	68%	18ml	0.27	2.7
冰醋酸	CP	1.8ml	0.032	0.32
水	纯水	35ml	1.94	19.44

2. 实验操作　在装有搅拌器、温度计、回流冷凝管和真空滴液漏斗的 150ml 四颈烧瓶中，依次加入水杨酸 13.8g 和水 35ml，加热搅拌至 50℃，固体全溶（附注 1）。搅拌下，缓慢滴加 68% 硝酸 18ml 和冰醋酸 1.8ml 的混合液（附注 2）。滴加完毕后，升温至 70 ~ 80℃，

反应约 2 小时。停止反应，将反应液倒入 120ml 冰水中，5℃放置 4 小时，析出固体，过滤，滤饼用冰水洗，得到 5 - 硝基水杨酸粗品。

将 5 - 硝基水杨酸粗品用热水重结晶，干燥得到淡黄色固体，即为 5 - 硝基水杨酸（8 - 2）。

3. 附注

（1）如果固体未全溶，可再加少许水使其溶解。

（2）实验中使用混酸硝化，反应剧烈，滴加混酸的速度不宜太快。可用冰水浴进行冷却控制硝化反应温度。

4. 思考题

（1）如何控制硝化反应条件？

（2）除了混酸外，还有哪几种常用的硝化试剂？

（二）美沙拉嗪的制备

1. 原料规格及配比 见表 8 - 2。

表 8 - 2 原料规格及配比表

原料名称	规格	用量	摩尔数	摩尔比
5 - 硝基水杨酸（附注）	自制	6.1g	0.033	1
还原铁粉	CP	9g	0.16	4.8
浓盐酸	CP	3ml	0.1	3
保险粉	AR	0.67g	0.004	0.12
水	纯水	35ml	1.97	59

2. 实验操作 在装有搅拌器、回流冷凝管和温度计的三颈烧瓶中，加入浓盐酸 3ml 和水 35ml，用油浴加热至 60℃，加铁粉 2.3g，加热回流 3 ~ 4 分钟。投入 5 - 硝基水杨酸约 1.5g，剧烈搅拌 5 分钟后，将剩余的 5 - 硝基水杨酸约 4.6g 及铁粉 6.7g 按上述的方式分三次加入，每次间隔 5 分钟。升温至 100℃反应 1.5 小时，停止反应，趁热用 50% 氢氧化钠溶液调节 pH 11 ~ 12，抽滤，滤饼用水洗两次，每次 10ml。滤液中加入保险粉 0.67g，用 40% 硫酸酸化至 pH 3 ~ 4。冷却析出固体，抽滤，干燥即得粗品 3g。

重结晶：取装有回流冷凝管的 100ml 圆底烧瓶，加入粗品 3g 溶于 35ml 热水中，加入亚硫酸氢钠 0.33g，活性炭 0.67g，加热回流 5 分钟，趁热过滤，热水洗涤，合并滤液和洗液。迅速冷却至 5℃，保温 1 小时后取出过滤，冰水洗涤两次，干燥，得白色针状结晶 2.5g。测熔点，计算收率。

3. 附注 根据实际得到的 5 - 硝基水杨酸的量，按表 8 - 2 所示比例计算各自的反应投料。

4. 思考题

（1）在本实验中，保险粉起什么作用？

（2）硝基的还原还可以采用哪些还原方法？并加以比较。

【美沙拉嗪的结构表征】

熔点：280℃。

^{1}H - NMR：结构正确（附图 8 - 1、附图 8 - 2）。

HRMS（ESI$^+$）：154.0471（M + H$^+$）（附图 8 - 3）。

HPLC 纯度：99.99%。

HPLC 测试的色谱条件：

色谱柱：十八烷基硅烷键合硅胶，Hypersil ODS（150mm × 4.0mm，5μm）。

流速：1.0ml/min。

进样量：10μl。

检测波长：254nm。

柱温：35℃。

流动相：以水（用磷酸调节 pH 至 2.5）- 甲醇（75 ： 25）为流动相。使用前需超声脱气。

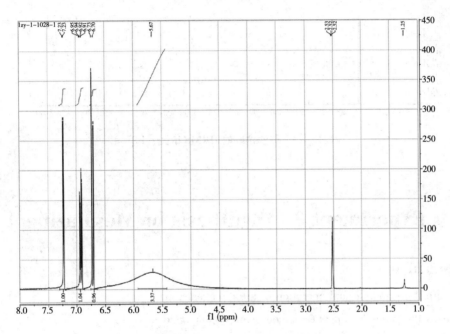

附图 8-1　美沙拉嗪的 ^{1}H - NMR 谱图（DMSO - d$_6$）

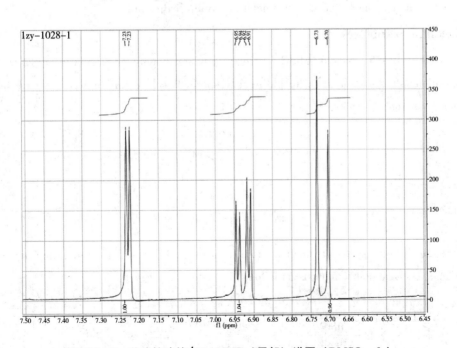

附图 8-2　美沙拉嗪的 ^{1}H - NMR（局部）谱图（DMSO - d$_6$）

Sample Name		Position	p1c1	Instrument Name	Instrument 1	User Name		G6520B−PC\Admin
Inj Vol	0.05	InjPosition		SampleType	Sample	IRM Calibration Status		Success
Data Filename	1zy−p.d	ACQ Method	20110418−MSonly−p.m	Comment		Acquired Time		10/28/2019 7:08:15 PM

$\times 10^6$ +ESI Scan(rt:0.244 min)Frag=120.0V 1zy−p.d Subtract(2)

154.0471

附图 8 − 3　美沙拉嗪的 HRMS 谱图（ESI⁺）

Experiment 8　Synthesis of Mesalazine

Experimental aim

1. Learn the principle and operation of nitration reaction.

2. Learn the general reductive method of nitro compound.

3. Learn the physico − chemical properties of mesalazine.

4. Learn the component and use of rongalite(sodium hydrosulfite).

Experimental principles

Mesalazine, alias:5 − amino salicylic acid, is a white to pink crystals with mp. 279 ~ 281℃ (decomposition). It is soluble in hydrochloric acid, sparingly soluble in hot water, slightly soluble in cold water or ethanol.

5 − amino − 2 − hydroxybenzoic acid

There are various synthetic methods formesalazine, one of which is nitration reduction of salicylic acid. The reaction formula is as follows：

70

Pre – lab preparation

1. Review the nitration reaction in organic chemistry and its reaction mechanism.

2. Learn the nitro reduction reaction in drug synthesis.

3. Learn physicochemical properties of mesalazine.

Knowledge point

Set – up of reaction apparatus, adding procedures of chemical reagents, nitration reaction, nitro reduction reaction, purity check.

Experiment procedures

Ⅰ. Preparation of 5 – nitro salicylic acid(8 – 2)

1. Materials(Table 8 – 1)

Table 8 – 1　Specification and ratio of raw materials

Materials	Specifications	Amount	Mol	Mol ratio
Salicylic acid(8 – 1)	Medicinal	13.8g	0.1	1
Concentratednitric acid	CP,68%	18ml	0.27	2.7
Glacial acetic acid	CP	1.8ml	0.032	0.32
Water	Pure water	35ml	1.94	19.44

2. Procedures　To a 150ml four – necked flask equipped with a stirrer, a refluxing condenser, a thermometer and a dropping funnel, salicylic acid 13.8g and water 35ml are added in turn. The reaction mixture is stirred and heated to 50℃ to dissolve salicylic acid(Note 1). A mixed solution of concentrated nitric acid 18ml and glacial acetic acid 1.8ml is added dropwise(Note 2). After addition of the mixed solution of nitric acid, the reaction temperature is raised to 70 ~ 80℃, and the temperature is maintained for 2h. The reaction mixture is poured into 120ml of ice – water, and the resultant mixture is kept at 5℃ for 4h. A solid is deposited. The precipitate is collected by suction and washed with ice – cold water, and a crude product of 5 – nitro salicylic acid is obtained.

After the above crude product is recrystallized with hot water, 5 – nitro salicylic acid(8 – 2) is obtained as a light – yellow crystal.

3. Notes

Note 1: If the solid can't be dissolved completely, some additional water should be added.

Note 2: A mixed acid is used as nitrating agent in this experiment. The dropping rate of mixed acid should be slow in order to avoid reacting tempestuously. An ice – bath could be used to control the reaction temperature.

4. Questions

(1) How to control thereaction conditions of nitration?

(2) Except mixed nitric acid, how many nitrating agents can be used for nitration reaction?

Ⅱ. Preparation of Mesalazine

1. Materials(Table 8-2)

Table 8-2　Specification and ratio of raw materials

Materials	Specifications	Amount	Mol	Mol ratio
5-nitro salicylic acid(8-2)(Note)	Obtained in last step	6.1g	0.033	1
Iron powder	CP	9g	0.16	4.8
Concentrated hydrochloric acid	CP	3ml	0.1	3
Rongalite(sodium hydrosulfite)	AR	0.67g	0.004	0.12
Water	Pure water	35ml	1.97	59

2. Procedures

To a 150ml four-necked flask equipped with a stirrer, a refluxing condenser and a thermometer, concentrated hydrochloric acid 3ml and water 35ml are added. The reaction mixture is heated to 60℃ with an oil-bath, and iron powder 2.3g is added, stirred and refluxed for 5min, and then 5-nitro salicylic acid 1.5g is added and stirred vigorously for 5min. The remanent 5-nitro salicylic acid 4.6g and iron powder 6.7g are divided into three portions and added by means of repeating above process every 5min. After addition of materials, the reaction temperature is raised to 100℃ and stirred for 1.5h. The pH of reaction mixture is adjusted to 11~12 with 50% sodium hydroxide while it is warm. The hot mixture is filtered and the filter cake is washed two times with water(10ml each time). Rongalite(sodium hydrosulfite)0.67g is added to the filtrate, and the pH of filtrate is adjusted to 3~4 with 40% sulfuric acid. The mixture is cooled and the precipitate is collected by suction, dried to give about 3g of crude product of mesalazine.

Recrystallization: To a 100ml round-bottom flask equipped with a refluxing condenser, 3g of crude product of mesalazine, 35ml of water and sodium bisulfite 0.33g are added, and the mixture is heated. After the solid dissolves, 0.67g of activated carbon is added and the mixture is heated and refluxed for 5min. The hot mixture is filtered and washed with hot water. The filtrate and washing solution are combined and cooled quickly to 5℃, and maintained for 1h. The precipitate is collected by suction and washed two times with ice-cold water, dried to give about 2.5g of mesalazine as a white-needle crystal. Measure the melting point and calculate the yield.

3. Notes

Note: Weigh the quantity of 5-nitro salicylic acid obtained by oneself, and calculate the inventory rating according to the ratio in Table 8-2.

4. Questions

(1) What effect does rongalite(sodium hydrosulfite) work in this experiment?

(2) What are the other reducing methods that could be used to reduce nitro group? Please compare them.

【Characterization of Mesalazine】

Melting point: 280℃.

^{1}H-NMR: Conformed(Attached figure 8-1 and 8-2).

HRMS(ESI$^+$): 154.0471(M+H$^+$)(Attached figure 8-3).

HPLC purity:99.9%.

HPLC conditions:

Column:C18,Hypersil ODS(150mm×4.0mm,5μm).

Flow rate:1.0ml/min.

Injection volume:10μl.

Detection wavelength:254nm.

Column temperature:35℃.

Mobile phase:Water(regulating pH value with phosphoric acid to 2.5)－methanol(75∶25)as mobile phase. Ultrasonic degassing before use.

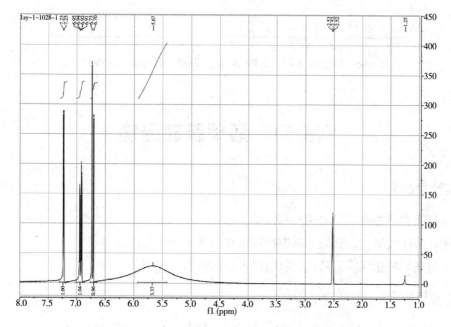

Attached figure 8－1 ¹H－NMR spectrum of mesalazine(DMSO－d₆)

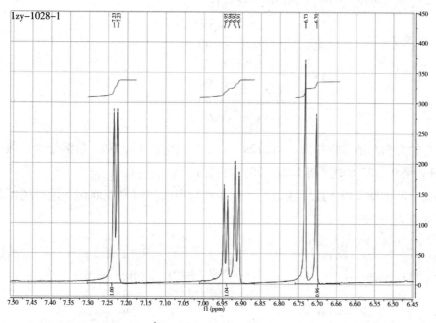

Attached figure 8－2 ¹H－NMR spectrum of mesalazine(DMSO－d₆)

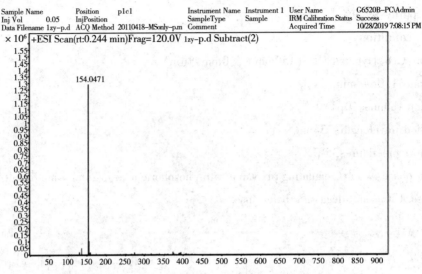

Attached figure 8 – 3   HRMS spectrum of mesalazine（ESI⁺）

实验九   葡甲胺的合成

【实验目的】

1. 通过实验熟悉高压釜的结构和性能。

2. 通过实际的操作，熟悉并掌握加压氢化的基本操作和注意事项。

3. 了解还原胺化反应的特点、机制以及反应终点的控制。

【实验原理】

葡甲胺（N – methylglucamine）化学名为 1 – 脱氧 – 1 –（甲氨基）– D – 山梨醇，［1 – deoxy – 1 – methylaminosorbitol］。化学结构式为：

$$
\begin{array}{c}
CH_2NHCH_3 \\
H \rule{1cm}{0.4pt} OH \\
HO \rule{1cm}{0.4pt} H \\
H \rule{1cm}{0.4pt} OH \\
H \rule{1cm}{0.4pt} OH \\
CH_2OH
\end{array}
$$

该化合物为白色结晶性粉末，mp. 129 ~ 131℃，密度为 1.375。易溶于水，微溶于乙醇（在 100ml 乙醇中，25℃时可溶 1.2g，70℃时可溶 21g）。

目前葡甲胺的制备以下述路线为主。葡萄糖与甲胺在雷尼镍催化下进行还原胺化一步反应得到葡甲胺。

$$
\begin{array}{c}
CHO \\
H \rule{1cm}{0.4pt} OH \\
HO \rule{1cm}{0.4pt} H \\
H \rule{1cm}{0.4pt} OH \\
H \rule{1cm}{0.4pt} OH \\
CH_2OH
\end{array}
+ CH_3NH_2
\xrightarrow[C_2H_5OH]{\text{雷尼镍; 15kg/cm}^2}
\begin{array}{c}
CH_2NHCH_3 \\
H \rule{1cm}{0.4pt} OH \\
HO \rule{1cm}{0.4pt} H \\
H \rule{1cm}{0.4pt} OH \\
H \rule{1cm}{0.4pt} OH \\
CH_2OH
\end{array}
$$

【实验预习】

1. 试述葡萄糖与甲胺在催化剂作用下进行还原胺化的反应过程。
2. 还原胺化反应的机制是什么？常用的还原剂又有哪些？
3. 使用加压氢化釜的操作流程以及需要注意的问题是什么？

【知识点】

仪器装置，投料过程，还原胺化，高压釜，催化剂，雷尼镍（Raney - Ni），重结晶，脱色，纯度检测。

【实验步骤】

（一）雷尼镍的制备

1. 原料规格及配比　见表 9 - 1。

表 9 - 1　原料规格及配比表

原料名称	规格	用量	摩尔数	摩尔比
铝镍合金	CP	50g	0.58	1
氢氧化钠	CP	50g	1.25	2.2
蒸馏水		200ml		
乙醇	95%	150ml		

2. 实验操作（附注 1）　在 800ml 烧杯中，加入氢氧化钠 50g 及蒸馏水 200ml，搅拌溶解。在水浴上加热到 50～85℃，搅拌下分批加入铝镍合金 50g（附注 2），约 45 分钟加完。再在 85～100℃搅拌 30 分钟，静置使镍沉降，倾去上层清液。以倾泻法用蒸馏水洗涤至中性，再用 95% 乙醇（每次 50ml）洗涤三次（附注 3），检查活性后用乙醇覆盖备用（附注 4）。

3. 附注

（1）雷尼镍的制备原理：氢氧化钠和铝镍合金中的铝反应，生成氢气和氢氧化铝，而留下蜂窝状的金属镍，在蜂窝状的金属镍表面吸附有残留氢气，成为雷尼镍催化剂。因此在整个实验中，应避免明火，以防着火发生事故。

（2）铝镍合金粉末含镍为 40%～50%。一次不宜加得过多，否则，会因反应剧烈产生很多气泡而溢出。

（3）在制备过程中严禁雷尼镍与自来水接触。

（4）本方法制备得到的是高活性的雷尼镍。

4. 思考题

（1）在制备雷尼镍催化剂时，为什么不能使用自来水？

（2）雷尼镍催化剂是如何分类的？常用的有哪几种？

（二）甲胺醇溶液的制备

1. 原料规格及配比　见表9-2。

表9-2　原料规格及配比表

原料名称	规格	用量	摩尔数	摩尔比
甲胺水溶液	CP	500ml	0.58	
95%乙醇	CP	480ml		

2. 实验操作　在1000ml的锥形瓶（吸收瓶）中放置95%乙醇480ml。在装有回流冷凝管的1000ml的圆底烧瓶（蒸发瓶）中放置甲胺水溶液500ml。

小心加热圆底烧瓶，使甲胺缓慢蒸发，甲胺气体通过回流冷凝器顶端导入装有固体氢氧化钠的干燥塔，干燥后进入吸收瓶吸收。当蒸发瓶中甲胺水溶液温度上升到92℃时，停止蒸馏，测定甲胺醇溶液的甲胺含量（附注），应在15%以上。若含量不足继续通甲胺，浓度过高则加入计算量的乙醇稀释到15%。

3. 附注　甲胺的含量测定：精密吸取1ml甲胺醇溶液于100ml容量瓶中，加水至刻度，摇匀。吸取20ml置于锥形瓶中，加40ml 0.1mol/L HCl标准溶液及酚酞指示液数滴。用0.1mol/L NaOH溶液滴定到显红色不退为止。

$$甲胺含量\% = \frac{N_{HCl} \times V_{HCl} - N_{NaOH} \times V_{NaOH} \times 0.03106}{1 \times 20/100} \times 100\%$$

（三）葡甲胺的制备

1. 原料规格及配比　见表9-3。

表9-3　原料规格及配比表

原料名称	规格	用量	摩尔数	摩尔比
葡萄糖	药用	6.0g	0.033	1
15%甲胺乙醇溶液	自制	29g	0.14	4.2
Raney - Ni	自制	1.3g		
95%乙醇	CP	150ml		
EDTA	CP	0.5g		

2. 实验操作　在100ml高压釜中，投入葡萄糖6g（附注1）、15%甲胺乙醇溶液29g及Raney - Ni 1.3g，再用少量乙醇冲洗附着在釜壁上的Raney - Ni。仔细地盖上釜盖，逐步对称地拧紧螺帽。按规定顺序排除釜内空气（附注2）。通氢气使釜内压力达到15kg/cm^2，关闭进气阀，启动搅拌，待正常后开始加热，维持温度在68℃±2℃。随时观察釜内压力变化，当压力降到10kg/cm^{2}时，补充氢气到15kg/cm^2。如此反复通氢气至氢压不再变化为止，约需6小时。停止搅拌，冷却至室温，打开排气阀排尽釜内残余空气，拧松螺帽，移开釜盖，吸出物料，过滤除去触媒（附注3）。滤液冷却到5℃以下，析出结晶，抽滤，得葡甲胺粗品。

粗品用6~8倍量蒸馏水溶解，加少量活性炭及0.5g EDTA的水溶液，加热回流，过滤，滤液在搅拌下慢慢倒入适量的乙醇中。冷却到5℃，析出结晶，抽滤，烘干后约得3g精制葡甲胺，收率46.2%。mp.128~131℃。

3. 附注

（1）一般用药用葡萄糖，经50~55℃干燥24小时后备用。

（2）高压釜中排除空气的操作步骤：拧开进气阀，通入氢气到 3kg/cm²，关闭进气阀，经检查无漏气现象后拧松排气阀，将气体放出（可稍留一些压力以防空气倒灌），关闭排气阀后重复以上操作两次，使高压釜中的空气全部排除，最后通入氢气至所需压力（15kg/cm²），拧紧进气阀，关闭钢瓶阀门，进行氢化。

（3）反应后的 Raney–Ni 催化剂仍有相当的活性，过滤时切勿滤干，以防催化剂燃烧。并立即用少量乙醇洗涤 3 次，然后将潮湿的触媒滤渣连同滤纸移到盛有乙醇的烧杯中回收。

4. 思考题

（1）在加压还原胺化反应中甲胺的摩尔比要过量很多，为什么？

（2）加压还原胺化反应要用何种压力表，能否用氧气压力表代替？

【葡甲胺的结构表征】

熔点：129～131℃。

^{1}H–NMR：结构正确（附图 9–1）。

MS（ESI^{+}）：196.3（M＋H^{+}）（附图 9–2）。

HPLC 纯度：99.8%。

HPLC 测试的色谱条件：

色谱柱：SHISEIDO SPOI AR C18。

流速：1.0ml/min。

进样量：20μg。

检测波长：195mm。

柱温：25℃。

流动相：乙腈–磷酸盐缓冲液（5∶95）。使用前需超声脱气。

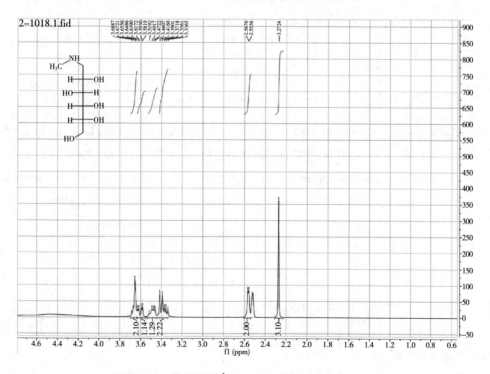

附图 9–1　葡甲胺的 ^{1}H–NMR 谱图（DMSO–d$_{6}$）

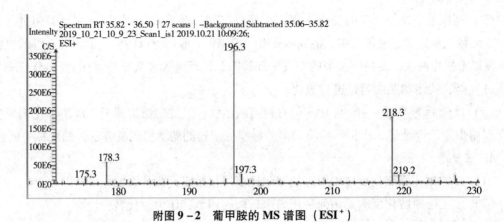

附图 9－2　葡甲胺的 MS 谱图（ESI⁺）

Experiment 9　　Synthesis of Methylglueamine

Experimental aim

1. Learn the construction and function of autoclave.

2. Learn the operation of hydrogenation under pressure.

3. Understand the process and mechanism of reductive amination.

Experimental principles

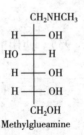

Methylglueamine

1 – Deoxy – 1 – methylaminosorbitol

Methylglueamine is a white crystalline powder with mp. 129 ~ 131℃. It is freely soluble in water, slightly soluble in ethanol(at 25℃ ,1. 2g/100ml EtOH；at 70℃ ,21g/100ml EtOH).

Methylglueamine is synthesized from glucose by reductive amination reaction with methylamine under catalysis of Raney – nickel. The synthetic route for methylglueamine is as follows：

$$
\text{glucose} + CH_3NH_2 \xrightarrow[\text{C}_2\text{H}_5\text{OH}]{\text{Raney–Ni; 15kg/cm}^2} \text{methylglueamine}
$$

Pre – lab preparation

1. Learn the reductive amination procedure of glucose with methylamine under catalysis of Raney – nickel.

2. Summerymechanism of the reductive amination and the common reductive reagents could be used.

3. Learn the operation process and precautions of pressure autoclave.

Knowledge point

Set – up of reaction apparatus, adding procedures of chemical reagents, reductive amination reaction, autoclave, catalysts, Raney – Ni, operation of recrystallization, purity test

Experiment procedures

Ⅰ. Preparation of Raney – Ni

1. Materials(Table 9 – 1)

Table 9 – 1　Specification and ratio of raw materials

Materials	Specifications	Amount	Mol	Mol ratio
Aluminum – nickel alloy	CP	50g	0.58	1
Sodium hydroxide	CP	50g	1.25	2.2
Distilled water		200ml		
95% ethanol	95%	150ml		

2. Procedures(Note 1)　To a 800ml beaker equipped with a stirrer, sodium hydroxide 50g and distilled water 200ml are added. The solution is heated to $50 \sim 85℃$ with stirring by a water – bath. Aluminum – nickel alloy 50g is added in several batches(Note 2). The total time for addition of aluminum – nickel alloy is about 45min. The reaction mixture is stirred for 30min at $85 \sim 100℃$, and then cooled to room temperature. The mixture is standing to settle nickel and the upper liquid is discarded. The nickel is washed with distilled water until the discarded water layer shows pH 7, and then it is washed three times with 95% ethanol(50ml each time)(Note 3). The resultant Raney – Ni is stored in ethanol after testing its activity(Note 4).

3. Notes

Note 1: The preparation principle of Raney – Ni: Sodium hydroxide reacts with aluminum in aluminum nickel alloy to generate hydrogen and aluminum hydroxide, leaving cellular nickel metal, adsorbing residual hydrogen on the surface of cellular nickel metal, which becomes Raney Ni catalyst. During the experiment, open fire must be avoided in case of the fire accident.

Note 2: Nickel content of aluminum – nickel alloy is about $40\% \sim 50\%$. Aluminum – nickel alloy should be added slowly, otherwise the aluminum – nickel alloy will react intensively with sodium hydroxide, which will give off a lot of bubbles, and cause the reaction mixture to overflow from the beaker.

Note 3: During the preparation process, it is strictly forbidden for Raney – Ni to touch with tap water.

Note 4: The high activity of Raney – Ni can be prepared from this method.

4. Questions

(1) Why is tab water not used in preparation of Raney – Ni catalysts?

(2) How about Raney – Ni catalysts classification and which are the common ones?

II. The preparation of alcoholic methylamine solution

1. Materials (Table 9 – 2)

Table 9 – 2 Specification and ratio of raw materials

Materials	Specifications	Amount	Mol	Mol ratio
Methylamine aqueous solution	CP	500ml	0.58	
95% ethanol	CP	480ml		

2. Procedures To a 1000ml erlenmeyer flask (absorption bottle, to absorb methylamine), 95% ethanol 480ml is placed. To a 1000ml round – bottom flask (distilling flask) equipped with a refluxing condenser, methylamine aqueous solution 500ml is placed.

The round – bottom flask contained methylamine aqueous solution is heated slowly to evaporate methylamine which passes through the refluxing condenser, and then passes through drying tower which is filled with solid sodium hydroxide, the dried methylamine enters into the absorption bottle in the end. When the temperature of methylamine aqueous solution in the flask rises to 92℃, the heating is stopped. The methylamine concentration of alcoholic methylamine solution is detected and the content of methylamine in alcohol should be more than 15% (Notes).

If themethylamine content is less than 15%, more methylamine aqueous solution in distilling flask should be evaporated, and more methylamine should be absorbed into ethanol in absorption bottle.

If the methylamine content is much more than 15%, a calculated ethanol should be added to adjust the methylamine content is 15%.

3. Notes Assay of the methylamine content: Transfer 1ml of alcoholic methylamine solution accurately to a 100ml volumetric flask. Add about 80ml of deionized water, and mix. Shake for a moment, dilute with deionized water to volume, and mix. Transfer 20ml of this solution to a conical flask, add 40ml of standard solution of 0.1mol/L hydrochloric acid and a few of drops of phenolphthalein indicators. Titrate hydrochloric acid against a standard solution of 0.1mol/L sodium hydroxide to a permanent light pink endpoint.

$$\text{Methylamine contents\%} = \frac{N_{\text{HCl}} \times V_{\text{HCl}} - N_{\text{NaOH}} \times V_{\text{NaOH}} \times 0.03106}{1 \times 20/100} \times 100\%$$

III. The preparation of methylglueamine

1. Materials (Table 9 – 3)

Table 9 – 3 Specification and ratio of raw materials

Materials	Specifications	Amount	Mol	Mol ratio
Glucose	medicinal	6.0g	0.033	1
15% alcoholic methylamine solution	prepared in last step	29g	0.14	4.2
Raney – Ni	prepared above	1.3g		
95% ethanol	CP	150ml		
EDTA	CP	0.5g		

2. Procedures To a 100ml autoclave, glucose 6g (Note 1), 15% alcoholic methylamine

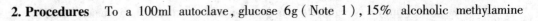

solution 29g and Raney – Ni 1.3g are added in turn, then the Raney – Ni clinging to the wall of autoclave is rinsed to the autoclave by a small quantity of ethanol. The autoclave – lid is closed with carefully, and the cap is fastened with nuts screwed symmetrically one by one. According to the proper order, the air in the autoclave is exhausted (Note 2) and the autoclave is full of hydrogen gas. The process of exhausting air and filling hydrogen is repeated for another two times. At last step, the hydrogen pressure of autoclave is filled to $15kg/cm^2$. Close gas admittance valve and turn on the stirrer. When the autoclave works normally, it is heated and maintained at $68℃ ±2℃$. More attention need be paid to the pressure. When the pressure is below $10kg/cm^2$, hydrogen gas is filled up again to $15kg/cm^2$, and this process is done repeatedly until the pressure in autoclave becomes invariableness. About 6h later, the reaction should complete. The stirrer is stopped, and the reaction mixture is cooled to room temperature. The exhaust valve is opened to release the remnant hydrogen gas. The nut is loosen and the lid is removed, and the reaction mixture is transfer to a flask by suction, and then filtered to remove catalyst (Note 3). The filtrate is cooled below $5℃$, a crude product of methylglueamine is collected by suction.

The crudeproduct is dissolved in $6 \sim 8$ times quantity of distilled water, and small quantity of activated carbon and EDTA 0.5g in water are added. The mixture is heated to reflux, and then filtered. The filtrate is poured slowly into a stirring ethanol. The mixture is cooled to $5℃$, and the resultant crystal is collected by suction and dried to give 3g of pure methylglueamine. The yield is about 46.2%, mp. $128 \sim 131℃$.

3. Notes

Note 1: Glucose is medicinal, which is previously dried at $50 \sim 55℃$ for 24h.

Note 2: The procedure of removing air from autoclave: Open gas admittance valve, press hydrogen gas into autoclave to a pressure of $3kg/cm^2$, close gas admittance valve. After examining whether any gas leaks from the autoclave, loosen slowly exhaust valve to release the gas (keeping a little pressure to avoid air flowing backwards). Close exhaust valve and repeat above operation twice to exhaust all of the air in autoclave, and then press hydrogen gas into autoclave until the pressure reaches $15kg/cm^2$. Close gas admittance valve and cylinder valve, and begin hydrogenation reaction.

Note 3: Raney – Ni in the reaction mixture is still active. It should be kept the Raney – Ni on filter paper in wet to avoid the catalyst self – ignite, when the reaction mixture is filtered. When the filtration is completed, Raney – Ni on filter paper should be washed thrice with ethanol immediately, and then the wet filter residue and filter paper are transferred into a beaker filled with ethanol.

4. Questions

(1) The mole number of methylamine is more than that of glucose in the reductive amination under high pressure, why?

(2) Which pressure gauge is used in the reductive amination under high pressure? Whether it could be replaced by oxygen pressure gauge?

【Characterization of Methyglueamine】

Melting point: $129 \sim 131℃$.

^{1}H – NMR：Conforms（Attached figure 9 – 1）.

MS（ESI$^+$）：196. 3（M + H$^+$）（Attached figure 9 – 2）.

HPLC：99. 8%.

HPLC conditions：

Column：SHISEIDO SPOI AR C18.

Flow rate：1. 0ml/min.

Injection volume：20μg.

Detection wavelength：195mm.

Column temperature：25℃.

Mobile phase：Acetonitrile – phosphate buffer（5：95）.

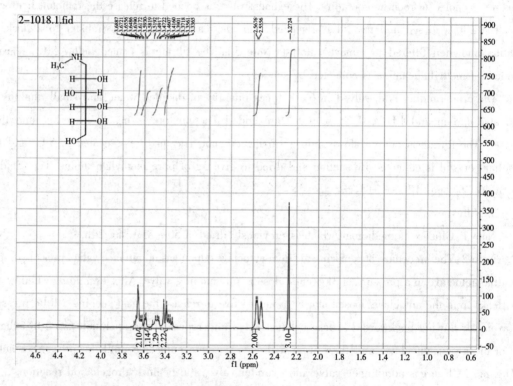

Attached figure 9 – 1 ^{1}H – NMR spectrum of methylglueamine（DMSO – d$_6$）

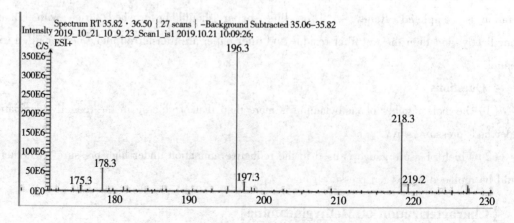

Attached figure 9 – 2   MS spectrum of methylglueamine（ESI$^+$）

实验十　兰索拉唑的合成

【实验目的】

1. 通过兰索拉唑的合成，熟悉缩合、氧化等反应。
2. 掌握兰索拉唑的精制方法。
3. 通过本实验，复习萃取、重结晶等基本操作。

【实验原理】

兰索拉唑（lansoprazole）的化学名为 2 -［［［3 - 甲基 - 4 -（2，2，2 - 三氟乙氧基）- 2 - 吡啶基］甲基］亚硫酰基］-1H - 苯并咪唑，［2 -［(RS) -［［3 - methyl - 4 -（2，2，2 - trifluoroethoxy）pyridin - 2 - yl］methyl］sulfinyl］-1H - benzimidazole］。化学结构式为：

兰索拉唑为白色或类白色结晶性粉末；mp. 178 ~ 182℃，遇光及空气易变质。在 N，N - 二甲基甲酰胺中易溶，在甲醇中溶解，在乙醇中略溶，在水中几乎不溶。

兰索拉唑的主要合成路线为：2 - 氯甲基 - 3 - 甲基 - 4 -（2，2，2 - 三氟乙氧基）吡啶盐酸盐（10 - 1）和 2 - 巯基苯并咪唑（10 - 2）发生缩合反应，得到中间体（10 - 3），然后经间氯过氧苯甲酸氧化、中和、淬灭得到兰索拉唑粗品，最后由乙醇重结晶得到兰索拉唑精品。

【实验预习】

1. 兰索拉唑的合成方法有哪些？各自有什么优缺点？
2. 该合成路线中缩合与氧化的机制是什么？还可以有哪些缩合、氧化方法？它们各自有什么优缺点？

3. 萃取和重结晶操作有哪些注意点？

【知识点】

仪器装置，投料过程，缩合反应，氧化反应，酸碱调节，萃取，重结晶，纯度检查。

【实验步骤】

（一）2－［［［3－甲基－4－（2，2，2－三氟乙氧基）－2－吡啶基］甲基］硫基］－1H－苯并咪唑（10－3）的合成

1. 原料规格及配比　表10－1所示。

表10－1　原料规格及配比表

原料名称	规格	用量	摩尔数	摩尔比
2－氯甲基－3－甲基－4－（2，2，2－三氟乙氧基）吡啶盐酸盐（10－1）	工业品	10g	0.036	1
2－巯基苯并咪唑（10－2）	工业品	6.5g	0.043	1.2
NaOH	CP	2.9g	0.072	2
甲醇	CP	100ml		
水	自来水	50ml		

2. 实验操作　在装有搅拌器、温度计及回流冷凝管的四颈瓶中，分别加入2－氯甲基－3－甲基－4－（2，2，2－三氟乙氧基）吡啶盐酸盐（10－1）、2－巯基苯并咪唑（10－2）、甲醇100ml，搅拌均匀后，加入氢氧化钠2.9g，升温至回流反应2.5小时，冷却到室温。冷至室温，过滤，蒸除滤液中的甲醇至总体积剩余约1/3（附注1），加水50ml（附注2），析出固体，室温搅拌30分钟，过滤，滤饼用水洗涤，干燥至恒重。得固体10.8g，收率84.4%。

3. 附注

（1）反应结束后需要蒸除大部分甲醇，如果甲醇剩余过多，产物损失大。

（2）应缓慢往甲醇中滴加水，防止析晶过快，包裹杂质。

4. 思考题　反应过程中的主要杂质是什么？是如何形成的？

（二）兰索拉唑粗品的制备

1. 原料规格及配比　见表10－2。

表10－2　原料规格及配比表

原料名称	规格	用量	摩尔数	摩尔比
中间体Ⅲ	自制	10.8g	0.030	1
间氯过氧苯甲酸	工业品	5.8g	0.033	1.1
乙酸乙酯	CP	108ml		

2. 实验操作　在装有搅拌器、温度计、恒压滴液漏斗及回流冷凝管的四颈瓶中，加入中间体（10－3）10.8g和乙酸乙酯50ml，冰盐浴保持在－5～0℃，滴加间氯过氧苯甲酸的

乙酸乙酯溶液（5.8g/58ml），40分钟内滴加完毕（附注1）。−5~0℃继续反应10分钟，反应结束后加入50ml 10%碳酸钠溶液，分出水层，有机层加入2g连二亚硫酸钠的30ml水溶液（附注2），合并水层，再加入30ml水萃取有机层一次，分出有机层。合并前三次水层后，用乙酸乙酯（20ml×3）反萃，合并所有有机层。减压浓缩，蒸去大部分乙酸乙酯，剩余10~15ml溶液冷却至−5~0℃析晶1小时，抽滤，少量乙酸乙酯洗滤饼，干燥至恒重，得到8.4g固体，收率75.0%。

3. 附注

（1）滴加间氯过氧苯甲酸时放热明显，需注意控制温度和滴加速度。

（2）氧化反应结束后，需要先用还原剂，如连二亚硫酸钠淬灭剩余的间氯过氧苯甲酸之后再进行后处理。

4. 思考题

（1）该氧化反应除了间氯过氧苯甲酸之外，还可以采用哪些氧化剂？

（2）如何减少过度氧化产物（即砜）的量？

（3）反应后处理还可以采用哪些还原剂进行淬灭？

（三）兰索拉唑的精制

1. 原料规格及配比 见表10-3。

表10-3 原料规格及配比表

原料名称	规格	用量	摩尔数	摩尔比
兰索拉唑粗品	自制	8.4g		
无水乙醇	CP	67.2ml		

2. 实验操作 往干燥的250ml单口瓶中加入8.4g兰索拉唑粗品、67.2ml无水乙醇，升温至回流使完全溶解，趁热过滤，滤液在0~5℃搅拌析晶2小时，抽滤，得产物，50℃真空干燥至恒重，得产物7.1g，收率84.5%，HPLC测得纯度99.9%。

3. 附注 重结晶操作时，需要趁热过滤去除不溶物。

4. 思考题 怎么选择重结晶的溶剂体系？

【兰索拉唑的结构表征】

熔点：178~182℃。

^{1}H−NMR：结构正确（附图10-1）。

HRMS（ESI$^+$）：370.0463（M+H$^+$）（附图10-2）。

HPLC纯度：99.9%。

HPLC测试的色谱条件：

色谱柱：十八烷基硅烷键合硅胶（4.6mm×250mm，5μm，或效能相当的色谱柱）。

流速：1.0ml/min。

进样量：10μl。

检测波长：284nm。

流动相：甲醇−水−三乙胺−磷酸（600∶400∶5∶1.5）[用磷酸溶液调节pH至7.3]。使用前需超声脱气。

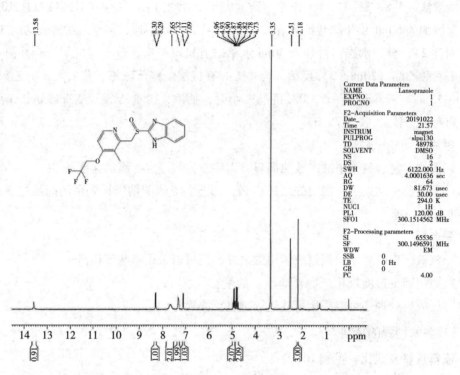

附图 10 – 1　兰索拉唑的 ^{1}H – NMR 谱图（DMSO – d_6）

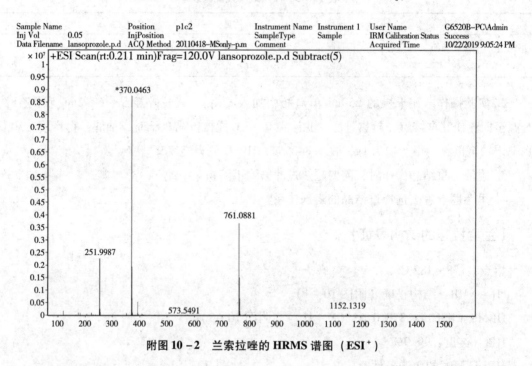

Sample Name		Position	p1c2	Instrument Name	Instrument 1	User Name	G6520B–PC\Admin
Inj Vol	0.05	InjPosition		SampleType	Sample	IRM Calibration Status	Success
Data Filename	lansoprozole.p.d	ACQ Method	20110418–MSonly–p.m	Comment		Acquired Time	10/22/2019 9:05:24 PM

附图 10 – 2　兰索拉唑的 HRMS 谱图（ESI$^+$）

Experiment 10　Synthesis of Lansoprazole

Experimental aim

1. Understand the condensation reaction and oxidation reaction through the synthesis

of lansoprazole

2. Learn the purification method of lansoprazole.

3. Review the operation of extraction and recrystallization.

Experimental principles

Lansoprazole

2 – [(RS) – [[3 – methyl – 4 – (2,2,2 – trifluoroethoxy)

pyridin – 2 – yl] methyl] sulfinyl] – 1H – benzimidazole

Lansoprazole is a white or off – white crystalline powder with mp. 178 ~ 182°C. It is easily deteriorated under light and in air. It is freely soluble in N,N – dimethylformamide, soluble in methanol, sparingly soluble in ethanol, and practically insoluble in water.

The main synthesis route of lansoprazole is as follow. 2 – (chloromethyl) – 3 – methyl – 4 – (2,2,2 – trifluoroethoxy) pyridine hydrochloride (10 – 1) is condensed with $1H$ – benzo [d] imidazole – 2 – thiol (10 – 2) to obtain an intermediate (10 – 3), which is then oxidized by m – chloroperoxybenzoic acid, neutralized, and quenched to obtain crude lansoprazole. Lansoprazole is finally recrystallized from ethanol to obtain purified lansoprazole.

(10–1)   (10–2)   (10–3)

Crude lansoprazole   Purified lansoprazole

Pre – lab preparation

1. Summarize the synthesis methods of lansoprazole and give a evaluate their advantages and disadvantages.

2. Analyze the mechanism of the condensation reaction and the oxidation reaction in this route. Please give out the other methods for these two reactions and evaluate their advantages and disadvantages.

3. What should be payed more attention in the operation of extraction and recrystallization?

Knowledge point

Set – up of reactionapparatus, adding procedures of chemical reagents, condensation reaction, oxidation reaction, acid – base adjustment, recrystallization, extraction, purity test.

Experiment procedures

Ⅰ. Synthesis of 2 – (((3 – methyl – 4 – (2, 2, 2 – trifluoroethoxy) pyridin – 2 – yl) methyl) thio) – 1H – benzo[d]imidazole(10 – 3)

1. Materials(Table 10 – 1)

Table 10 – 1　Specification and ratio of raw materials

Materials	Specifications	Amount	Mol	Mol ratio
2 – (chloromethyl) – 3 – methyl – 4 – (2, 2, 2 – trifluoroethoxy) pyridine hydrochloride(10 – 1)	Industrialgrade	10g	0. 036	1
1H – benzo[d]imidazole – 2 – thiol(10 – 2)	Industrialgrade	6. 5g	0. 043	1. 2
NaOH	CP	2. 9g	0. 072	2
Methanol	CP	100ml		
H_2O	Natural water	50ml		

2. Procedures　2 – (chloromethyl) – 3 – methyl – 4 – (2, 2, 2 – trifluoroethoxy) pyridine hydrochloride(10 – 1), 1H – benzo [d] imidazole – 2 – thiol (10 – 2) and methanol 100ml were added successively to a four – necked flask equipped with stirrer, thermometer and condenser. The mixture was stirred at room temperature to form a solution. Then NaOH 2. 9g was added to the solution, and the mixture was heated to reflux for 2. 5 hours. After the end of the reaction, the mixture was cooled to room temperature, and then filtered. The filtrate was concentrated to remove 2/ 3 of methanol(Note 1). 50ml of water was added to the residual(Note 2). The residual mixture was cooled and filtered. The filtrate cake was washed by water, and then dried to constant weight. 10. 8 of solid was obtained, and the yield is 84. 4%.

3. Notes

Note 1: The majority of the methanol in the filtrate should be removed by distillation under reduced pressure, otherwise, the yield is low.

Note 2: Water should be added slowly to the methanol residual to prevent impurities wrapped in the deposited product.

4. Questions　What is the main impurityin this reaction process and how dose it form?

Ⅱ. Synthesis of crude lansoprazole

1. Materials(Table 10 – 2)

Table 10 – 2　Specification and ratio of raw materials

Materials	Specifications	Amount	Mol	Mol ratio
2 – (((3 – methyl – 4 – (2, 2, 2 – trifluoroethoxy) pyridin – 2 – yl) methyl) thio) – 1H – benzo[d] imidazole(10 – 3)	Prepared in last step	10. 8g	0. 030	1
m – chlorobenzoperoxoic acid	Industrial grade	5. 8g	0. 033	1. 1
Ethyl acetate	CP	108ml		

2. Procedures 2 – (((3 – methyl – 4 – (2,2,2 – trifluoroethoxy) pyridin – 2 – yl) methyl) thio) – 1H – benzo[d]imidazole(10 – 3)10. 8g and ethyl acetate 50ml were added successively to a four – necked flask equipped with stirrer, thermometer, constant pressure dropping funnel and condenser. The flask was cooled with an ice brine bath to keep the temperature between – 5℃ to 0℃. m – chlorobenzoperoxoic acid 5. 8g in ethyl acetate 58ml was added dropwise slowly into the flask during 40min from the constant pressure dropping funnel(Note 1). The reaction mixture was continually stirred for 10min at – 5℃ to 0℃. After the end of the reaction, 10% sodium carbonate solution 50ml was added (Note 2). The water layer was separated and the organic layer was extracted respectively with $Na_2S_2O_4$ solution($Na_2S_2O_4$ 2g in water 30ml) and water 30ml. Then, three parts of water layers were combined, and treated with of ethyl acetate(20ml × 3). The all organic layers were combined, and concentrated to 10 ~ 15ml under reduced pressure. The concentrated solution was stood for crystallization. The crystal was collected by filtration and the filtrate cake was washed by ethyl acetate. Crude lansoprazole solid 8. 4g was obtained, and the yield is 75. 0%.

3. Notes

Note 1: When m – chloroperoxybenzoic acid is added dropwise, the heat release is obvious. It is necessary to control the temperature and dropping speed.

Note 2: After the end of the oxidation reaction, the remained m – chloroperoxybenzoic acid should be quenched firstly with a reducing agent such as sodium dithionite.

4. Questions

(1)Which oxidants could be used in this oxidation reaction, except m – chloroperoxybenzoic acid?

(2)How to reduce the amount of excessive oxidation products(ie. sulfones)?

(3)What other reducing agents can be used for quenching m – chloroperoxybenzoic acid after the reaction?

Ⅲ. Purification of Lansoprazole

1. Materials(Table 10 – 3)

Table 10 – 3　Specification and ratio of raw materials

Materials	Specifications	Amount	Mol	Mol ratio
Crude lansoprazole	Prepared in last step	8. 4g		
Ethanol	CP	67. 2ml		

2. Procedures Crude lansoprazole 8. 4g was dissolved in ethanol 67. 2ml. The solution was heated to reflux until it becomes clear. Then the solution was filtered while hot(Notes). The filtrate was stood for crystallization with stirring under 0 ~ 5℃ for 2 hours. The crystal was collected by filtering and washed by ethanol. The crystal was dried and 7. 1g lansoprazole was obtained, yield 84. 5%, purity 99. 9% by HPLC.

3. Notes　The hot filtration is necessary to remove the insoluble matter.

4. Questions How to choose a solvent system forrecrystallization?

【Characterization of Lansoprazole】

Melting point:178 ~ 182℃.

^{1}H – NMR:Conforms(Attached figure 10 – 1).

HRMS(ESI^{+}):370. 0463(M + H^{+})(Attached figure 10 – 2).

HPLC purity:99. 9%.

HPLC conditions:

Column:C18(4. 6mm × 250mm,5μm).

Flow rate:1. 0ml/min.

Injection volume:10μl.

Detection wavelength:284nm.

Mobile phase:Methanol – water – triethylamine – phosphoric acid(600 : 400 : 5 : 1. 5),adjust to pH = 7. 3 with phosphoric acid. Ultrasonic degassing before use.

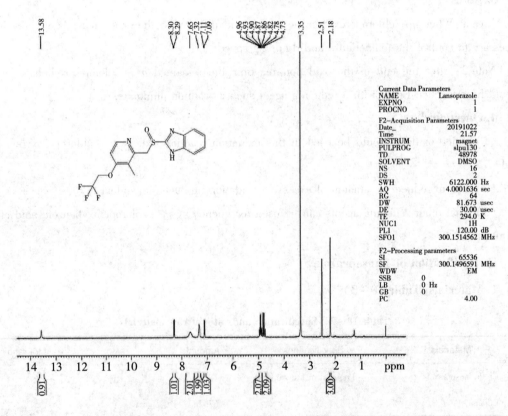

Attached figure 10 – 1 ^{1}H – NMR spectrum of lansoprazole(DMSO – d$_{6}$)

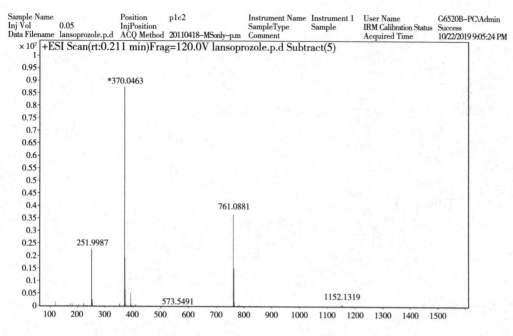

Sample Name		Position	p1c2	Instrument Name	Instrument 1	User Name	G6520B–PC\Admin
Inj Vol	0.05	InjPosition		SampleType	Sample	IRM Calibration Status	Success
Data Filename	lansoprozole.p.d	ACQ Method	20110418–MSonly–p.m	Comment		Acquired Time	10/22/2019 9:05:24 PM

Attached figure 10 – 2 HRMS spectrum of lansoprazole (ESI +)

实验十一 那格列奈的合成

【实验目的】

1. 通过那格列奈的合成实验，熟悉酰胺制备的一般方法。

2. 通过实验，掌握减压浓缩和重结晶的操作。

【实验原理】

那格列奈（nateglinide），化学名 N –（反式 – 4 – 异丙基环己基 – 1 – 甲酰基）– D – 苯丙氨酸，[N –（trans – 4 – isopropylcyclohexyl – 1 – carbonyl）– D – phenylalamine]。化学结构式为：

Nateglinide

那格列奈为白色或类白色结晶性粉末，mp. 为 137 ~ 141℃。在甲醇、乙醇、三氯甲烷中易溶，在丙酮、乙醚中溶解，水中几乎不溶。

那格列奈的合成路线是以苯丙氨酸（11 – 1）为原料，与甲醇成酯（11 – 2）后和反式 – 4 – 异丙基环己基甲酸（11 – 3）在二环己基碳二亚胺（DCC）催化下缩合，得到那格列奈甲酯（11 – 4），最后水解得到那格列奈。

91

那格列奈

【实验预习】

1. 试述 D - 苯丙氨酸和甲醇反应生成甲酯的反应过程。

2. DCC 在酰胺缩合过程中起了什么作用？是否可以用其他试剂替代？

3. 重结晶的具体目的是什么？重结晶的溶剂该怎样选择？

【知识点】

仪器装置，酯的合成，酰胺的合成，缩合剂，重结晶，酸碱调节，纯度检查，TLC 操作。

【实验步骤】

（一） D - 苯丙氨酸甲酯（11 - 2）的合成

1. 原料规格及配比　见表 11 - 1。

表 11 - 1　原料规格及配比表

原料名称	规格	用量	摩尔数	摩尔比
D - 苯丙氨酸（11 - 1）	CP	2.6g	0.0156	1
氯化亚砜	CP	5.7ml	0.0796	5
甲醇	CP	20ml		

2. 实验操作　向 100ml 三颈瓶中加入 D - 苯丙氨酸（11 - 1）2.6g，甲醇 20ml（附注 1），搅拌条件下降温至 0℃，缓慢滴加氯化亚砜 5.7ml（附注 2）。滴加完毕后，撤去冰浴，室温搅拌 1 小时。减压浓缩（附注 3），得白色固体 3.31g，计算收率。

3. 附注

（1）甲醇应事先处理为无水甲醇，否则氯化亚砜会被甲醇中微量水分解。

（2）在滴加氯化亚砜的过程中须保持反应液温度低于 5℃。

（3）减压浓缩时需防止水倒吸至反应瓶中。如发生水倒吸时，剩余的氯化亚砜遇水分解放出大量的 HCl 和 SO_3 气体，需密切注意。

4. 思考题

（1）是否有其他合成苯丙氨酸甲酯的方法？

（2）实验中在使用氯化亚砜时需要注意什么？

（二）那格列奈甲酯（11-4）的合成

1. 原料规格及配比 见表11-2。

表11-2 原料规格及配比表

原料名称	规格	用量	摩尔数	摩尔比
D-苯丙氨酸甲酯（11-2）	CP	3.2g	0.0147	1
反式-4-异丙基环己基甲酸（11-3）	CP	2.5g	0.0147	1
二环己基碳二亚胺（DCC）	CP	3.3g	0.0161	1.1
三乙胺	CP	1.6g	0.0161	1.1
二氯甲烷	CP	35ml		

2. 实验操作 在250ml三颈瓶内加入D-苯丙氨酸甲酯（11-2）3.2g，反式-4-异丙基环己基甲酸（11-3）2.5g，二氯甲烷25ml，室温搅拌。于搅拌状态下加入三乙胺1.6g，加毕，将反应液降温至0℃，慢慢滴加二环己基碳二亚胺（DCC）3.3g的二氯甲烷（10ml）溶液，滴加完毕，室温反应10小时。抽滤，滤液减压浓缩，得粗品4.51g。将粗品用甲醇20ml重结晶（附注），得白色固体3.9g，计算收率。

3. 附注 重结晶时，甲醇用量不宜过多，以到达回流温度时，粗品恰好溶解为最佳。

4. 思考题 DCC在反应后，自身生成的产物是什么？如何去除？

（三）那格列奈的制备

1. 原料规格及配比 见表11-3。

表11-3 原料规格及配比表

原料名称	规格	用量	摩尔数	摩尔比
那格列奈甲酯（11-4）	自制	3.9g	0.0118	
2mol/L氢氧化钠溶液		25ml		
甲醇	CP	25ml		
浓盐酸	CP	适量		

2. 实验操作 向250ml的三颈瓶中，加入那格列奈甲酯（11-4）3.9g，2mol/L氢氧化钠水溶液25ml，甲醇25ml，室温搅拌2小时。抽滤，滤液减压蒸除甲醇，残余液用浓盐酸（附注）调节pH至2左右，抽滤，滤饼干燥后得白色固体那格列奈2.1g，计算收率，熔点：137～141℃，HPLC纯度：99.8%。

3. 附注 调节pH的过程中，须在冰浴条件下进行，缓慢滴加浓盐酸。使用浓盐酸的过程中注意防护。

4. 思考题 酯水解过程中，碱的种类和浓度如何选择？

【那格列奈的结构表征】

熔点：137～141℃。

^{1}H - NMR：结构正确（附图 11 - 1）。

HRMS（ESI$^+$）：340.0（M + Na$^+$）（附图 11 - 2）。

HPLC 纯度：99.8%。

HPLC 测试的色谱条件：

色谱柱：Symmetry C18（4.6mm × 250mm，5μm）。

流速：1.0ml/min。

进样量：10μl。

检测波长：214nm。

柱温：室温。

流动相：乙腈 - 磷酸盐（取磷酸二氢钾 4.08g 溶解于 900ml 水中，用磷酸调节 pH 2.8，再用水稀释至 1000ml）（41∶59）。使用前需超声脱气。

理论塔板数大于 3000。

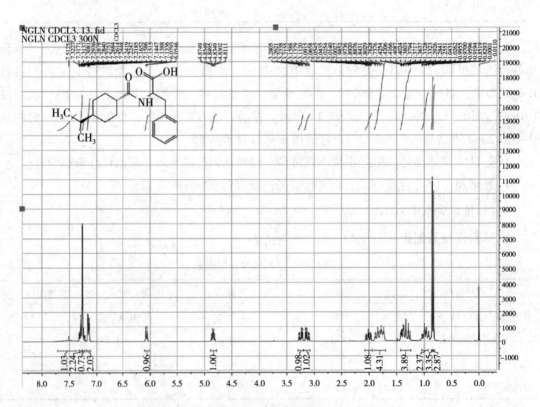

附图 11 - 1　那格列奈的^{1}H - NMR 谱图（CDCl$_3$）

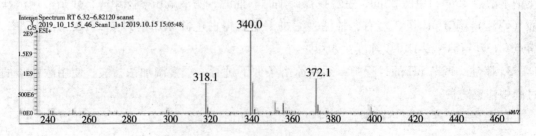

附图 11 - 2　那格列奈 HRMS 谱图（ESI$^+$）

Experiment 11   Synthesis of Nateglinide

Experimental aim

1. Get preliminary knowledge of generalpreparation method of amide through the synthesis of nateglinide.

2. Train the basic experimentaloperation of vacuum concentration and recrystallization in this experiment.

Experimental principles

Nateglinide

$N -($ trans $- 4 -$ isopropylcyclohexyl $- 1 -$ carbonyl $) -$ D $-$ phenylalamine

Nateglinide is a white or crystalline power with mp. $137 \sim 141\,^{\circ}\mathrm{C}$. It is freely soluble in methanol, ethanol and chloroform, soluble in acetone and ether and practically insoluble in water.

The synthesis process of nateglinide is shown as follow: D – phenylalanine (11 – 1) was converted to methyl D – phenylalaninate hydrogen chloride (11 – 2) in methanol and $SOCl_2$. Then, (11 – 2) condensed with *trans* – 4 – isopropylcyclohexane – 1 – carboxylic acid (11 – 3) to produce nateglinide methyl ester (11 – 4) by catalysis of N, N' – dicyclohexylcarbodiimide (DCC). Nateglinide methyl ester was hydrolyzed with sodium hydroxide to produce nateglinide.

Nateglinide

Pre – lab preparation

1. Discuss the reaction process of D – phenylalanine with methanol to form methyl D – phenylalaninate.

2. Review the role of DCC in the amide condensation process and discuss wether DDC could be

95

substituted by other condensation reagents.

3. Discuss the purpose and specific steps of recrystallization. How to choose the solvent for recrystallization?

Knowledge point

Set – up of reaction apparatus, adding procedures of chemical reagents, recrystallization, acid – base adjustment, purity test, TLC operation.

Experiment procedures

Ⅰ. The preparation of methylphenylalaninate hydrogen chloride(11 – 2)

1. Materials(Table 11 – 1)

Table 11 – 1　Specification and ratio of raw materials

Materials	Specifications	Amount	Mol	Mol ratio
D – phenylalanine(11 – 1)	CP	2.6g	0.0156	1
Thionyl chloride	CP	5.7ml	0.0796	5
Methanol	CP	20ml		

2. Procedures　To a 100ml three – necked flask, D – phenylalanine (11 – 1) 2.6g and methanol 20ml were added(Note 1), and the mixture was cooled to 0℃ with an ice bath by stirring, then thionyl chloride 5.7ml was slowly added dropwise(Note 2). After the dropwise addition was completed, the ice bath was removed and the mixture was stirred at room temperature for 1 hour. The reaction solution was concentrated under reduced pressure (Note 3) to give a white solid 3.31g. Calculated yield.

3. Notes

Note 1: Methanol should be pretreated for anhydrous, since thionyl chloride will be decomposed by trace water in methanol.

Note 2: The temperature of the reaction solution must be kept below 5℃ during the dropwise addition of thionyl chloride.

Note 3: It is necessary to prevent water from being sucked into the reaction bottle during vacuum concentration. In case of water reverse suction, the remaining thionyl chloride will decompose with water and release a large amount of HCl and SO_3 gas, which should be paid close attention to.

4. Questions

(1) Are there any other methods to synthesis of methylphenylalaninate?

(2) What should be notice when usethionyl chloride in experiment?

Ⅱ. The preparation of nateglinide methyl ester(11 – 4)

1. Materials(Table 11 – 2)

Table 11 – 2　Specification and ratio of raw materials

Materials	Specifications	Amount	Mol	Mol ratio
Methyl D – phenylalaninate hydrogen chloride (11 – 2)	Prepared in the last step	3.2g	0.0147	1

Continued

Materials	Specifications	Amount	Mol	Mol ratio
Trans – 4 – isopropylcyclohexane – 1 – carboxylic acid(11 –3)		2.5g	0.0147	1
DCC	CP	3.3g	0.0161	1.1
Triethylamine	CP	1.6g	0.0161	1.1
Methylene dichloride	CP	35ml		

2. Procedures　To a 250ml three – necked flask, methyl D – phenylalaninate hydrogen chloride(11 – 2) 3.2g, *trans* – 4 – isopropylcyclohexane – 1 – carboxylic acid (11 – 3) 2.5g, dichloromethane 25ml were added and stirred at room temperature. Triethylamine 1.6g was added under stirring. After the addition was completed, the reaction solution was cooled to 0℃ and DCC 3.3g in dichloromethane 10ml is added dropwise slowly. After the dropwise addition was completed, the reaction mixture was stirred at room temperature for 10 hours. The reaction mixture was filtrated with suction, and the filtrate was concentrated under reduced pressure to give a crude product. A crude product 4.51g was obtained and recrystallized with 20ml of methanol(Notes), to give a white solid 3.9g. Calculated yield.

3. Notes　In recrystallization, the amount of methanol should be controlled to just dissolve the crude product under reflux temperature and was not excess.

4. Questions　What will DCC become after reaction and how to remove it?

Ⅲ. The preparation of Nateglinide

1. Materials(Table 11 –3)

Table 11 –3　Specification and ratio of raw materials

Materials	Specifications	Amount	Mol	Mol ratio
Nateglinide methyl ester(11 –4)	Prepared in the last step	3.9g	0.0118	
2mol/L sodium hydroxide solution		25ml		
Methyl alcohol	CP	25ml		
Hydrochloric acid	CP	appropriate amount		

2. Procedures　To a 250ml three – necked flask, nateglinide methyl ester (11 – 4) 3.9g, 2mol/L sodium hydroxide solution 25ml, methanol 25ml were added and stirred at room temperature for 2h. The reaction mixture was filtrated with suction, and the methanol was removed under reduced pressure. The residue was adjusted to pH 2 with concentrated hydrochloric acid(Notes), and a solid was precipitated. The solid was collected by filtration and dried to give a white solid 3.2g (nateglinide), calculated yield.

3. Notes　The pH adjustment process must be carried out under ice bath conditions, and concentrated hydrochloric acid should be slowly added dropwise. Take care for yourself when using concentrated hydrochloric acid.

4. Questions　How to choosea base and its concentration for the ester hydrolysis?

【Characterization of Nateglinide】

Melting point：137～141℃.

^{1}H – NMR：Conforms（Attached figure 11 – 1）.

MS（ESI$^+$）：340. 0（M + Na$^+$）（Attached figure 11 – 2）.

HPLC purity：99. 8%.

HPLC conditions：

Column：Symmetry C18（4. 6mm×250mm,5μm）.

Flow rate：1. 0ml/min.

Injection volume：10μl.

Detection wavelength：214nm.

Mobile phase：Acetonitrile – phosphate（take potassium dihydrogen phosphate 4. 08g dissolved in 900ml water,adjust pH 2. 8 with phosphoric acid,dilute with water to 1000ml）（41∶59）；The number of theoretical plates is greater than 3000.

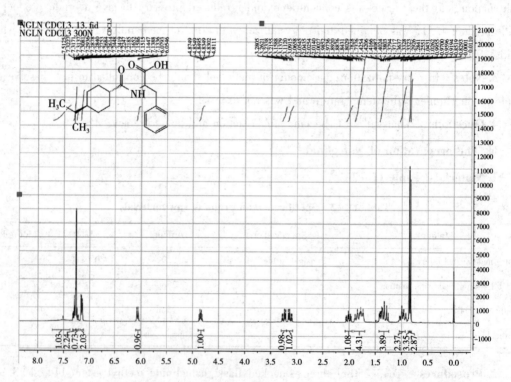

Attached figure 11 – 1 ^{1}H – NMR spectrum of nateglinide

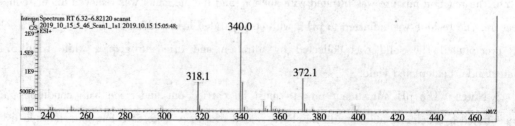

Attached figure 11 – 2   HRMS spectrum of nateglinide（ESI$^+$）

实验十二 厄贝沙坦的合成

【实验目的】

1. 了解厄贝沙坦的临床用途、工业生产及市场情况。
2. 通过厄贝沙坦的合成实验，掌握吉厄贝沙坦的合成方法。
3. 通过实际操作，学习原料药厄贝沙坦的精制方法。

【实验原理】

厄贝沙坦（irbesartan）的化学名为 2 – 丁基 – 3 – [4 – [2 – (1H – 四氮唑 – 5 – 基) 苯基] 苯甲基] – 1, 3 – 二氮杂螺 [4, 4] 壬 – 1 – 烯 – 4 – 酮，[2 – butyl – 3 – [[2′ – (1H – tetrazol – 5 – yl) biphenyl – 4 – yl] methyl] – 1, 3 – diazaspiro [4.4] non – 1 – en – 4 – one]。化学结构式为：

厄贝沙坦为白色或类白色粉或结晶性粉末，mp. 180 ~ 181℃。在甲醇或乙醇中微溶，在水中不溶。

厄贝沙坦的工业生产主要以以下路线为主：2 – 丁基 – 1, 3 – 二氮杂螺 [4, 4] 壬 – 1 – 烯 – 4 – 酮盐酸盐（12 – 1）和 5 – [4′ – (溴甲基) – (1, 1′ – 二苯基) – 2 – 基] – 1 – 三苯甲基 – 1H – 四氮唑（12 – 2）经缩合得到中间体 2 – 丁基 – 3 – [4 – [2 – (1 – 三苯甲基 – 1H – 四氮唑 – 5 – 基) 苯基] 苯甲基] – 1, 3 – 二氮杂螺 [4, 4] 壬 – 1 – 烯 – 4 – 酮（12 – 3），然后水解并成盐得到厄贝沙坦盐酸盐粗品（12 – 4），（12 – 4）经碳酸氢钠中和得到厄贝沙坦粗品，最后经乙醇重结晶得到厄贝沙坦精品。

厄贝沙坦粗品

厄贝沙坦精品

【实验预习】

1. 厄贝沙坦的合成方法有哪些？请对其优缺点进行评价。

2. 脱除三苯甲基保护基的方法有哪些？

3. 重结晶的目的是什么？具体的步骤包括哪些？

【知识点】

仪器装置，投料过程，烃化反应，重结晶，酸碱调节，保护基脱除，纯度检查，TLC 操作。

【实验步骤】

（一） 2 - 丁基 - 3 - [4 - [2 - (1 - 三苯甲基 - 1H - 四氮唑 - 5 - 基） 苯基] 苯甲基] - 1，3 - 二氮杂螺 [4，4] 壬 - 1 - 烯 - 4 - 酮（12 - 3） 的合成

1. 原料规格及配比 见表 12 - 1。

表 12 - 1 原料规格及配比表

原料名称	规格	用量	摩尔数	摩尔比
2 - 丁基 - 1，3 - 二氮杂螺 [4，4] 壬 - 1 - 烯 - 4 - 酮盐酸盐（12 - 1）	工业品	10.15g	0.044	1.1
5 - [4′ - (溴甲基) - (1，1′ - 二苯基) - 2 - 基] - 1 - 三苯甲基 - 1H - 四氮唑（12 - 2）	工业品	22.30g	0.040	1
KOH	CP	10.86g	0.194	4.6
四丁基溴化铵（$Bu_4N^+Br^-$）	CP	1.80g	0.005	0.14
甲苯	CP	78ml		
水	自来水	39ml		

2. 实验操作 在 250ml 三颈烧瓶中，依次加入甲苯 78ml、2 - 丁基 - 1，3 - 二氮杂螺 [4，4] 壬 - 1 - 烯 - 4 - 酮盐酸盐（12 - 1） 10.15g 、四丁基溴化铵（$Bu_4N^+Br^-$）1.80g 、 5 - [4′ - (溴甲基) - (1，1′ - 二苯基) - 2 - 基] - 1 - 三苯甲基 - 1H - 四氮唑（12 - 2）

22.30g，搅拌。另取 KOH 10.86g 溶解于水 39ml 中，缓慢滴加到反应瓶中（附注 1），加热回流反应 2 小时（附注 2），TLC 检测［展开剂 PE（石油醚）：EA（醋酸乙酯）= 5：1］反应完全，静置分层，甲苯层用水 39ml 洗涤（附注 3），减压蒸除甲苯，得黄色油状物，直接用于下一步反应。

3. 附注

（1）滴加 KOH 水溶液时有放热现象，需要缓慢滴加。

（2）反应液在升温之前为乳白色浑浊液体，加热至回流后，固体逐渐溶解至澄清。

（3）水洗涤时如果出现乳化，可以考虑加入饱和氯化钠水溶液，促其分层。

4. 思考题 反应过程中加入四丁基溴化铵（$Bu_4N^+Br^-$）的作用是什么？请列出几种可以替代四丁基溴化铵的试剂。

（二）厄贝沙坦盐酸盐（12-4）的合成

1. 原料规格及配比 见表 12-2。

表 12-2 原料规格及配比表

原料名称	规格	用量	摩尔数	摩尔比
2-丁基-3-[4-[2-(1-三苯甲基-1H-四氮唑-5-基）苯基］苯甲基]-1,3-二氮杂螺［4，4］壬-1-烯-4-酮（12-3）	自制	上一步油状物		
36% 浓盐酸	CP	11.8ml		
乙醇	CP	130ml		
水	自来水	130ml		

2. 实验操作 在 250ml 三颈烧瓶中，加入 2-丁基-3-[4-[2-(1-三苯甲基-1H-四氮唑-5-基）苯基］苯甲基]-1,3-二氮杂螺［4，4］壬-1-烯-4-酮（12-3）（上一步所得油状物）、无水乙醇 130ml。搅拌下，加入水 65ml，然后滴加 36% 的盐酸 11.8ml（5 分钟内加毕）（附注 1），在 15~25℃ 搅拌 2 小时，TLC 检测反应完全（展开剂同上）。抽滤去除滤饼，滤液减压蒸除大部分乙醇，加入水 65ml（附注 2）。继续在 15~25℃ 搅拌析晶 2 小时，抽滤，得白色固体，60℃ 干燥至干燥失重 ≤1.0%，得固体 19.58g。将该固体加入 250ml 三口烧瓶中，同时加入固体重量 2.5 倍体积的丙酮（约 49ml），加热回流 1 小时，冷却至 0~10℃，在该温度搅拌 2 小时，抽滤，滤饼 50℃ 真空干燥至干燥失重 ≤1.0%，得白色固体 14.45g，两步总产率 77.7%。

3. 附注

（1）浓盐酸需要滴加，不可以一次性加入，否则会有结块现象。

（2）减压蒸除乙醇后，需要在剧烈搅拌下缓慢加入水，否则会瞬间析出油状物，油状物固化后变硬，导致无法搅拌，且抽滤困难。

4. 思考题 反应结束后抽滤去除固体的主要成分是什么？

（三）厄贝沙坦（粗品）的制备

1. 原料规格及配比 见表 12-3。

表 12 - 3 原料规格及配比表

原料名称	规格	用量	摩尔数	摩尔比
厄贝沙坦盐酸盐（12 - 4）	自制	14.45g		
NaHCO₃	CP	适量		
无水乙醇	CP	86ml		
水	自来水	43ml		

2. 实验操作 在入 250ml 三口烧瓶中，依次加入无水乙醇 86ml 、水 43ml 和厄贝沙坦盐酸盐（12 - 4）14.45g，搅拌使固体溶解。在 15 ~ 25℃，所得溶液用饱和 NaHCO₃ 水溶液调节 pH 至 5.0 ~ 5.5（附注），析出大量晶体，继续搅拌 2 小时。抽滤，得到固体，60℃ 干燥至干燥失重≤1.0%，得白色固体 12.25g，产率 92.0%。

3. 附注 碳酸氢钠水溶液应缓慢滴加，如果滴加过快，析出的固体会包裹无机盐等杂质。

4. 思考题 是否可以使用碳酸钠或者氢氧化钠进行中和反应？

（四）厄贝沙坦的精制

1. 原料规格及配比 见表 12 - 4。

表 12 - 4 原料规格及配比表

原料名称	规格	用量	摩尔数	摩尔比
厄贝沙坦粗品	自制	12.25g		
无水乙醇	CP	122ml		

2. 实验操作 往干燥的 250ml 单口瓶中加入厄贝沙坦粗品 12.25g、无水乙醇 122ml，升温至回流使完全溶解，冷却至 70℃，加入 0.15g 活性炭（防止暴沸）（附注 1），回流 10 分钟，趁热抽滤去除活性炭（附注 2），滤液在 0 ~ 10℃ 搅拌析晶 4 小时，抽滤，得固体，在 50℃ 真空干燥至干燥失重≤0.5%，得产物 9.7g，收率 80.0%，HPLC 测得纯度 99.9%。

3. 附注

（1）加入活性炭之前需要先适当降温，防止暴沸。

（2）趁热过滤时，不可以一次性将反应液倒入布氏漏斗中，防止降温后产物在布氏漏斗上析出。

4. 思考题 重结晶为什么要加入活性炭？为什么要趁热过滤？

【厄贝沙坦的结构表征】

熔点：180 ~ 181℃。

¹H - NMR：结构正确（附图 12 - 1）。

HRMS（ESI⁺）：429.2404（M + H⁺）（附图 12 - 2）。

HPLC 纯度：99.9%。

HPLC 测试的色谱条件：

色谱柱：Diamonsil C18（150mm × 4.6mm，5μm）。

流速：1.0ml/min。

进样量：10μl。

检测波长：245nm。

柱温：35℃。

流动相：磷酸溶液（取 85% 磷酸 5.5ml，加水至 950ml，以三乙胺调节 pH 至 3.2）-乙腈（62：38）。使用前需超声脱气。

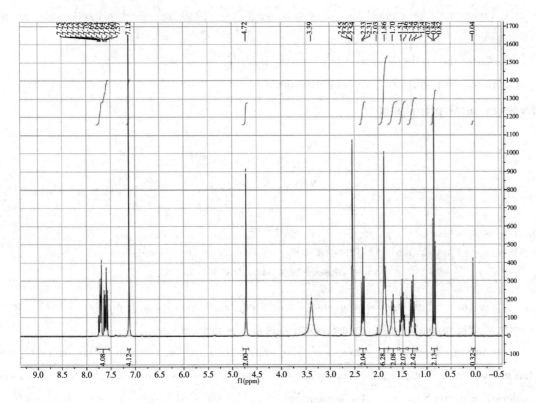

附图 12-1　厄贝沙坦的 ^1H-NMR 谱图（DMSO-d_6）

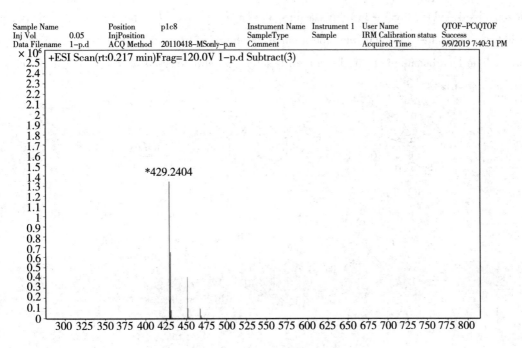

附图 12-2　厄贝沙坦的 HRMS 谱图（ESI$^+$）

Experiment 12   Synthesis of Irbesartan

Experimental aim

1. Understand the clinical use, industrialmanufacture procedures and market conditions of irbesartan.

2. Master the synthesis method of irbesartan from this experiment.

3. Learn the purification method of irbesartan

Experimental principles

Irbesartan

2 – butyl – 3 – [[2′ – (1H – tetrazol – 5 – yl) biphenyl – 4 – yl] methyl] – 1,

3 – diazaspiro [4,4] non – 1 – en – 4 – one

Irbesartan is white or off – white powder or a crystalline powder with mp. 180 ~ 181℃. It is slightly soluble in methanol or ethanol, and insoluble in water.

The industrial production process of irbesartan is mainly based on the following route: the starting material 2 – butyl – 1,3 – diazaspiro [4,4] non – 1 – en – 4 – one hydrochloride (12 – 1) is condensed with the 5 – (4′ – (bromomethyl) – [1,1′ – biphenyl] – 2 – yl) – 1 – trityl – 1H – tetrazole(12 – 2)to obtain 2 – butyl – 3 – ((2′ – (1 – trityl – 1H – tetrazol – 5 – yl) – [1,1′ – biphenyl] – 4 – yl) methyl) – 1,3 – diazaspiro [4,4] non – 1 – en – 4 – one(12 – 3), which is then hydrolyzed and salted to obtain the irbesartan hydrochloride (12 – 4), and (12 – 4) is neutralized with sodium bicarbonate to obtain the crude irbesartan, which is recrystallized from ethanol to obtain purified irbesartan.

$$\xrightarrow[\text{EtOH/H}_2\text{O}]{\text{NaHCO}_3}$$

（12-4）

$$\xrightarrow[\text{EtOH}]{\text{Activated carbon}}$$

Crude Irbesartan

Irbesartan

Pre – lab preparation

1. Summarize the all synthetic methods of irbesartan and give an evaluation of these methods for their advantages and disadvantages.

2. Discuss the all methods for deprotecting trityl group.

3. Review the purpose and specific steps of recrystallization.

Knowledge point

Set – up of reaction apparatus, adding procedures of chemical reagents, alkylation reaction, recrystallization, acid – base adjustment, protecting group removal, purity test, TLC operation.

Experiment procedures

Ⅰ. **Synthesis of 2 – butyl – 3 – ((2′ – (1 – trityl – 1H – tetrazol – 5 – yl) – [1,1′ – biphenyl] – 4 – yl)methyl) – 1,3 – diazaspiro[4,4]non – 1 – en –4 – one(12 –3)**

1. Materials(Table 12 –1)

Table 12 – 1　Specification and ratio of raw materials

Materials	Specifications	Amount	Mol	Mol ratio
2 – butyl – 1,3 – diazaspiro[4,4]non – 1 – en – 4 – one hydrochloride(12 – 1)	Industrial material	10. 15g	0. 044	1. 1
5 – (4′ – (bromomethyl) – [1,1′ – biphenyl] – 2 – yl) – 1 – trityl – 1H – tetrazole(12 – 2)	Industrial material	22. 30g	0. 040	1
KOH	CP	10. 86g	0. 194	4. 6
Bu$_4$N$^+$Br$^-$	CP	1. 80g	0. 005	0. 14
Toluene	CP	78ml		
H$_2$O	Tap water	39ml		

2. Procedures　To a 250ml three – necked flask, toluene 78ml, 2 – butyl – 1,3 – diazaspiro [4,4]non – 1 – en – 4 – one hydrochloride(12 – 1)10. 15g, Bu$_4$N$^+$Br$^-$ 1. 80g and 5 – (4′ –

105

(bromo methyl) – [1,1′ – biphenyl] – 2 – yl) – 1 – trityl – 1H – tetrazole 22. 30g were added successively. The mixture was stirred at room temperature. To another flask was added KOH 10. 86g and water 39ml. The KOH aqueous solution was added slowly to the above reaction mixture(Note 1), and then the mixture was heated to reflux for 2 hours(Note 2). After the end of the reaction monitored by TLC(PE(petroleum) : EA(ethyl acetate) = 5 : 1), the reaction mixture was stood for separation, the toluene layer was separated, and washed with water 39ml(Note 3). The organic layer was concentrated under reduced pressure and yellow oil was obtained.

3. Notes

Note 1:The addition of KOH solution is exothermic, so it should be added dropwise slowly.

Note 2:The reaction solution is a milky white turbid liquid before heating, and after heating to reflux, the solid gradually dissolves until clarification.

Note 3: A saturated aqueous solution of sodium chloride would be added in case of emulsification during extraction.

4. Questions What is the effect of $Bu_4N^+Br^-$ during the reaction? Please list several other reagents that can replace $Bu_4N^+Br^-$.

II. Synthesis of irbesartan hydrochloride(12 – 4)

1. Materials(Table 12 – 2)

Table 12 – 2   Specification and ratio of raw materials

Materials	Specifications	Amount	Mol	Mol ratio
2 – butyl – 3 – ((2′ – (1 – trityl – 1H – tetrazol – 5 – yl) – [1,1′ – biphenyl] – 4 – yl) methyl) – 1,3 – diazaspiro[4,4]non – 1 – en – 4 – one(12 – 3)	Prepared in last step	Oil obtained in the last step		
36% hydrochloricacid solution	CP	11. 8ml		
Ethanol	CP	130ml		
H_2O	Tap water	130ml		

2. Procedures   2 – Butyl – 3 – ((2′ – (1 – trityl – 1H – tetrazol – 5 – yl) – [1,1′ – biphenyl] – 4 – yl) methyl) – 1,3 – diazaspiro[4,4]non – 1 – en – 4 – one(12 – 3), the oil obtained in the last step and anhydrous ethanol 130ml were added to a 250ml three – necked flask, then water 65ml was added. The mixture was stirred and a 36% hydrochloric acid solution 11. 8ml were added dropwise slowly to the flask(in 5min)(Note 1). The reaction mixture was stirred at 15 ~ 25℃ for 2 hours. The end of the reaction was monitored by TLC(PE : EA = 5 : 1). The mixture was filtered, and the filtrate was concentrated under reduced pressure to remove most volume of ethanol. To the the raffinate, water 65ml was added with stirring(Note 2), and the reaction mixture was stirred for another 2 hours at 15 ~ 25℃. The mixture was filtered, and the cake was dried at 60℃ for 6 hours to obtain white solid 19. 58g. The white solid 19. 58 and 2. 5 times volume of acetone by weight of solid(about 49ml) were added to a 250ml three – necked flask, and the mixture was heated to reflux for 1 hour. Then the mixture was cooled to 0 ~ 10℃, and stirred for 2 hours at 0 ~ 10℃. The mixture was filtered. The cake obtained was dried under vacuum for 6 hours to obtain white solid 14. 45g. The overall yield of the two steps was 77. 7%.

3. Notes

Note 1: Concentrated hydrochloric acid solution should be added dropwise, otherwise, the irbesartan hydrochloride(12 - 4) produced will agglomerate.

Note 2: After removing most volume of ethanol under reduced pressure, water should be added under vigorous stirring, otherwise the oil will be precipitated immediately, and then solidifies and hardens, resulting in failure to stir, and difficulty in filtration.

4. Questions What is the main component of the solid removed by filtration after the end of the reaction?

Ⅲ. Preparation of crude irbesartan

1. Materials(Table 12 - 3)

Table 12 - 3 Specification and ratio of raw materials

Materials	Specifications	Amount	Mol	Mol ratio
Irbesartan Hydrochloride(12 - 4)	Prepared in last step	14.45g		
NaHCO$_3$	CP	Appropriate amount		
Ethanol	CP	86ml		
H$_2$O	Tap water	43ml		

2. Procedures To a 250ml three - necked flask, anhydrous ethanol 86ml, water 43ml and irbesartan hydrochloride(12 - 4)14.45g were added succesively and the mixture was stirred at 15 ~ 25℃ until the solution was clear. Then saturated NaHCO$_3$ aqueous solution was added slowly to the mixture to adjust to pH = 5.0 ~ 5.5(Notes), with precipitation of a great deal of crystals and the mixture was stirred for another 2 hours. Then, the mixture was filtered by suction, the cake was dried at 60℃ to obtain a white solid 12.25g. The yield was 92.0%.

3. Notes The sodium bicarbonate aqueous solution should be added dropwise slowly. Otherwise, the precipitated solid may wrap some impurities such as inorganic salts.

4. Questions Whether sodium carbonate or sodium hydroxide can be used for neutralization?

Ⅳ. Purification of irbesartan

1. Materials(Table 12 - 4)

Table 12 - 4 Specification and ratio of raw materials

Materials	Specifications	Amount	Mol	Mol ratio
Crude irbesartan	Prepared in last step	12.25g		
Ethanol	CP	122ml		

2. Procedures Crude irbesartan 12.25g obtained in the last step and anhydrous ethanol 125ml were heated to reflux in a 250ml three - necked flask, and the mixture become clear. Then the reaction temperature was decreased to 70℃, activated carbon 0.15g was added(Note 1), and the mixture was heated to reflux again for 10 minutes. The mixture was filtered by suction with hot to remove the active carbon(Note 2), and the filtrate was stirred at 0 ~ 10℃ for 4 hours, filtered, and the cake obtained was dried under vacuum for 5 hours at 50℃ to obtain white solid 9.7g, purity 99.9% by HPLC.

3. Notes

Note 1:Before adding activated carbon, it is necessary to cool down the mixture to prevent from bumping.

Note 2:During filtration with hot, the reaction solution should not be poured into the Buchner funnel at one time to prevent the product from being precipitated on the Buchner funnel after cooling.

4. Questions   Why activated carbon should be added during recrystallization? Why should we filter to remove active carbon with hot?

【Characterization of Irbesartan】

Melting point:180~181℃.

^1H-NMR:Conforms(Attached figure 12-1).

HRMS(ESI^+):429.2404($M+H^+$).

HPLC conditions:

Column:Diamonsil C18(150mm×4.6mm,5μm).

Flow rate:1.0ml/min.

Injection volume:10μl.

Detection wavelength:245nm.

Column temperature:35℃.

Mobile phase:Phosphoric acid solution(5.5ml of 85% phosphoric acid,dilute to 950ml with water,adjust to pH = 3.2 with triethylamine) – Acetonitrile(62:38). Ultrasonic degassing before use.

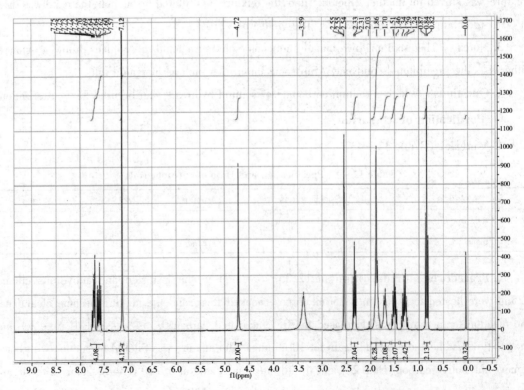

Attached figure 12-1 ^1H-NMR spectrum of irbesartan(DMSO-d_6)

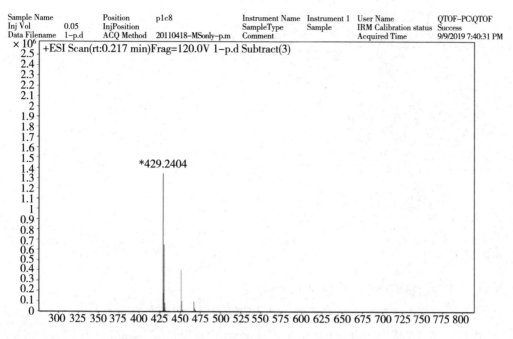

Sample Name
Inj Vol 0.05
Data Filename 1-p.d

Position p1c8
InjPosition
ACQ Method 20110418-MSonly-p.m

Instrument Name Instrument 1
SampleType Sample
Comment

User Name QTOF-PC\QTOF
IRM Calibration status Success
Acquired Time 9/9/2019 7:40:31 PM

+ESI Scan(rt:0.217 min)Frag=120.0V 1-p.d Subtract(3)

*429.2404

Attached figure 12 - 2　HRMS spectrum of irbesartan(ESI$^+$)

实验十三　吉非罗齐的合成

【实验目的】

1. 通过对吉非罗齐合成路线的比较，使学生掌握选择实际生产工艺的几个基本要求。

2. 通过实际操作，对涉及到的各类反应特点、机制、操作要求、反应终点的控制等，进一步巩固有机化学实验的基本操作，领会掌握理论知识。

3. 掌握各步中间体的质量控制方法。

【实验原理】

吉非罗齐（gemfibrozil）的化学名为 5 - (2，5 - 二甲基苯氧基) - 2，2 - 二甲基戊酸，[5 - (2，5 - dimethylphenoxy) - 2，2 - dimethylpentanoic acid]。化学结构式为：

吉非罗齐为白色结晶性粉末，mp. 61 ~ 63℃，几乎不溶于水，易溶于二氯甲烷，可溶于无水乙醇和甲醇。

吉非罗齐的制备方法很多，现选用一条较为简单的路线。由 2，5 - 二甲基苯酚（13 -1）与 1 - 溴 - 3 - 氯丙烷反应得到中间体 2 - (3 - 氯丙氧基) - 1，4 - 二甲基苯（13 - 2），再与异丙酸反应得到吉非罗齐。

吉非罗齐

【实验预习】

1. 烃化反应有哪些类型，各自的注意事项是什么？
2. 分析合成路线中的副产物有哪些，以及如何减少这些副产物的产生。
3. 吉非罗齐的合成方法有哪些？并对其优缺点进行评价。

【知识点】

仪器装置，投料过程，烃化反应，重结晶，萃取，纯度检查。

【实验步骤】

（一）2-（3-氯丙氧基）-1，4-二甲基苯（13-2）的制备

1. 原料规格及配比 见表13-1。

表13-1 原料规格及配比表

原料名称	规格	用量	摩尔数	摩尔比
2，5-二甲基苯酚（13-1）	工业品	7.5g	0.061	1
1-溴-3-氯丙烷	工业品	9.1ml	0.092	1.5
叔丁醇钾	CP	10.0g	0.092	1.5
无水四氢呋喃	CP	30+50ml		
乙醚	CP	30ml		
10% NaOH 水溶液	CP	120ml		
无水硫酸钠	CP			

2. 实验操作 在250ml三颈瓶中，放入1-溴-3-氯丙烷9.1ml和无水四氢呋喃30ml（附注），搅拌下滴加溶有2，5-二甲基苯酚（13-1）7.5g和叔丁醇钾10.0g的四氢呋喃（50ml）溶液，滴加完毕后升温至65℃，搅拌4小时。反应结束后，冷至室温。

减压蒸除四氢呋喃溶液，加入乙醚萃取（20ml×3），合并有机层用10% NaOH溶液洗涤（40ml×3）去除未反应的原料2，5-二甲基苯酚，无水硫酸钠干燥。有机层减压蒸馏，得棕黄色油状物。

3. 附注 本反应为无水反应，所有仪器应事先烘干。

4. 思考题 试比较常压蒸馏与减压蒸馏的原理、仪器和操作过程的不同之处。

（二）吉非罗齐的合成

1. 原料规格及配比 见表 13-2。

表 13-2 原料规格及配比表

原料名称	规格	用量	摩尔数	摩尔比
2-（3-氯丙氧基）-1，4-二甲基苯（13-2）	自制	5g	0.025	1
2mol/L 二异丙基氨基锂（LDA）的无水四氢呋喃溶液	CP	50ml	0.100	4
异丁酸	CP	5ml	0.055	2.2
无水四氢呋喃	CP	50ml		
水	CP	50ml		
乙醚	CP	180ml		
2mol/L HCl	自制			

2. 实验操作 将 2mol/L 二异丙基氨基锂（LDA）的无水四氢呋喃溶液 50ml 置于反应瓶中，在 0℃ 和 N_2 保护条件下缓慢加入异丁酸 5ml，冰浴下搅拌 2 小时，0℃ 冰浴条件下缓慢滴加溶有 2-（3-氯丙氧基）-1，4-二甲基苯（13-2）5g 的无水四氢呋喃（50ml）溶液，室温反应 5 小时。反应完毕后加入水 50ml 淬灭未反应的 LDA，分离去除有机层（附注）。

水层用乙醚洗涤（30ml×3），水相用稀 HCl 调节 pH 至 4~5，有白色絮状沉淀生成。水相用乙醚萃取（30ml×3），乙醚层无水硫酸钠干燥，减压蒸馏收集 158~159℃/2.67Pa 的馏分，并用己烷结晶，得吉非贝齐。

3. 附注 当水层中无机盐较多时，四氢呋喃与水混溶的比例会明显减小，可以分层。

4. 思考题 试分析二异丙基氨基锂的作用，是否可用其他试剂替换。

【吉非罗齐的结构表征】

熔点：61~63℃。

^1H-NMR：结构正确（附图 13-1）。

HRMS（ESI^+）：251.1644（$M+H^+$）（附图 13-2）。

HPLC 纯度：99.5%。

HPLC 测试的色谱条件：

色谱柱：十八烷基硅烷键合硅胶（4.6mm×150mm，5μm）。

流速：0.5ml/min。

进样量：10μl。

检测波长：245nm。

流动相：乙腈（加 0.1% 甲酸）：水 =9：1。使用前需超声脱气。

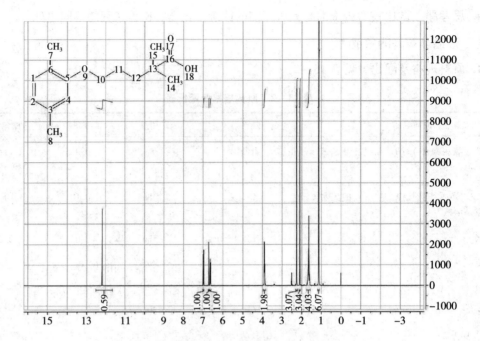

附图 13 – 1　吉非罗齐的 ^{1}H – NMR 谱图（DMSO – d_6）

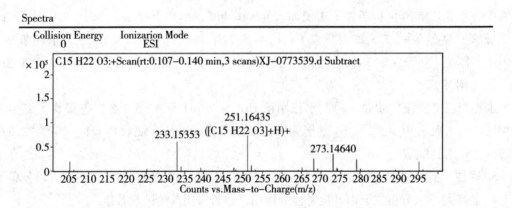

附图 13 – 2　吉非罗齐的 HRMS 谱图（ESI$^+$）

Experiment 13　Synthesis of Gemfibrozil

Experimental aim

1. Learn how to select a practical process on the basis of comparison of several different synthetic routes.

2. Understand the reaction characteristic, mechanism, operation requirement, control of reaction endpoint act and train the basic experimental operation skills of organic synthesis through the experiment.

3. Learn the quality control method of intermediates in every reaction step.

Experimental principles

$$5-(2,5-\text{dimethylphenoxy})-2,2-\text{dimethylpentanoic acid}$$

Gemfibrozil

Gemfibrozil is a white crystalline powder with mp. $61 \sim 63\,℃$. It is practically insoluble in water, freely soluble in dichloromethane, and soluble in anhydrous ethanol and methanol.

There are many preparation routes of gemfibrozil based on different starting materials. A simple process used in industrial manufacture of gemfibrozil over ten years is shown as follow.

2,5 – dimethylphenol(13 – 1) reacted with 1 – bromo – 3 – chloropropane to produce 2 – (3 – chloro propoxy) – 1,4 – dimethylbenzene(13 – 2). Then,(13 – 2) reacted with isobutyric acid to yield gemfibrozil.

Gemfibrozil

Pre – lab preparation

1. List the types of alkylation reaction and summerize the differences of these reaction.
2. Analyze what is the byproduct in this synthetic process and how to reduce the byproduct.
3. Evaluate the advantages and disadvantages of different synthetic routes of gemfibrozil.

Knowledge point

Set – up of reaction apparatus, adding procedures of chemical reagents, acylation reaction, recrystallization, operation of recrystallization and extraction, purity test.

Experiment procedures

Ⅰ. Synthesis of 2 – (3 – chloropropoxy) – 1,4 – dimethylbenzene(13 – 2)

1. Materials(Table 13 – 1)

Table 13 – 1　Specification and ratio of raw materials

Materials	Specifications	Amount	Mol	Mol ratio
2,5 – dimethylphenol(13 – 1)	Industrial Material	7.5g	0.061	1
1 – bromo – 3 – chloropropane	Industrial Material	9.1ml	0.092	1.5
Potassium t – butoxide	CP	10.0g	0.092	1.5

Continued

Materials	Specifications	Amount	Mol	Mol ratio
Anhydrous tetrahydrofuran	CP	30 + 50ml		
Ether	CP	30ml		
10% NaOH solution	CP	120ml		
Anhydrous sodium sulphate	CP			

2. Procedures　1 – bromo – 3 – chloropropane 9. 1ml and anhydrous tetrahydrofuran 30ml were added to a 250ml three – necked flask equipped with stirrer, condenser and thermometer (Notes). Then a mixture of 2,5 – dimethylphenol(13 – 1)7. 5g and potassium t – butoxide 10. 0g in anhydrous tetrahydrofuran 50ml were added slowly dropwise to the flask with stirring at room temperature. After dropping addition, the reaction mixture was stirred at 65℃ for 4h. After completion of reaction, the mixture was cooled to room temperature.

Tetrahydrofuran was removed by distillation in vacuum. Extraction the mixture with ether(20ml ×3) and the combined organic layer was washed with 10% sodium hydroxide solution(20ml × 3) to remove the unreacted 2,5 – dimethylphenol, dried with anhydrous sodium sulphate. A brown liquid was obtained by vacuum distillation.

3. Notes　This reaction was carried out under anhydrous environment and all glassware and flasks should be dried before use.

4. Questions　Compare and discuss the differences between atmospheric distillation and vacuum distillation.

Ⅱ. Synthesis of Gemfibrozil

1. Materials(Table 13 –2)

Table 13 –2　Specification and ratio of raw materials

Materials	Specifications	Amount	Mol	Mol ratio
2 – (3 – chloropropoxy) – 1,4 – dimethylbenzene(13 –2)	Self – prepared	5g	0. 025	1
2mol/L lithium diisopropylamide (LDA) in THF	CP	50ml	0. 100	4
Isobutyric acid	CP	5ml	0. 055	2. 2
Anhydrous tetrahydrofuran(THF)	CP	50ml		
Water	CP	50ml		
Ether	CP	180ml		
2mol/L HCl	Self – prepared			

2. Procedures　To a flask containing 2mol/L lithium diisopropylamide(LDA) in THF 50ml, isobutyric acid was slowly added at 0℃ under N_2 atmosphere protected. The mixture was stirred at 0℃ for 2 hours. The 2 – (3 – chloropropoxy) – 1,4 – dimethylbenzene(13 – 2)5g dissolved in anhydrous tetrahydrofuran 50ml was added to the above mixture at 0℃, the mixture was stirred at room temperature for another 5 hours. At last, water 50ml were added to the reaction mixture to quenching unreacted LDA. The organic layer was separated and removed(Notes).

The aqueous layer was washed by ether(30ml ×3) and acidified with HCl to adjust pH = 4 ~5. A white flocculent precipitation produced. Then the mixture was exacted with ether(30ml ×3), and the combined ether layer was dried with anhydrous sodium sulphate. Gemfibrozil was collected between 158 ~159℃/2. 67Pa by reduced pressure distillation, and was further recrystallized with hexane.

3. Notes The miscible proportion of tetrahydrofuran with water will decrease obviously, when more inorganic salts was dissolved in the water, and it will cause stratification of tetrahydrofuran with water.

4. Questions Please explain the effect of lithium diisopropylamide(LDA), and discuss if LDA could be replace by another reagents.

【Characterization of Gemfibrozil】

Melting point:61 ~63℃.

^{1}H - NMR:Conforms(Attached figure 13 - 1).

HRMS(ESI$^+$):251. 1644(M + H$^+$)(Attached figure 13 - 2).

HPLC purity:99. 5%.

HPLC conditions:

Column:C18(4. 6mm × 150mm,5μm).

Flow rate:0. 5ml/min.

Injection volume:10μl.

Detection wavelength:245nm.

Mobile phase:Acetonitrile(with 0. 1% formic acid) - Water(9 : 1). Ultrasonic degassing before use.

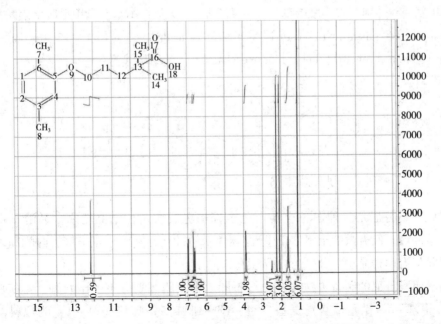

Attached figure 13 - 1 ^{1}H - NMR spectrum of gemfibrozil(DMSO - d$_6$)

Spectra

Collision Energy   Ionizarion Mode
0   ESI

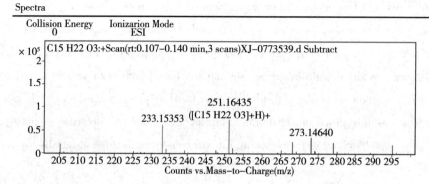

Attached figure 13 – 2   HRMS spectrum of gemfibrozil(ESI $^+$)

实验十四　甲磺酸伊马替尼的合成

【实验目的】

1. 了解伊马替尼的合成工艺研究和临床用途。
2. 了解药物晶型现象对药物性质的影响。
3. 掌握还原反应和缩合反应的基本原理和实验操作。
4. 掌握结晶及萃取等实验操作。

【实验原理】

甲磺酸伊马替尼（imatinib mesylate）的化学名为 4 – ［（4 – 甲基 – 1 – 哌嗪基）甲基］–
N –［4 – 甲基 – 3 – ［［4 –（3 – 吡啶基）– 2 – 嘧啶基］– 氨基］苯基］苯甲酰胺甲磺酸盐，［4 –
［（4 – methyl – 1 – piperazinyl）methyl］– N –［4 – methyl – 3 – ［［4 –（3 – pyridinyl）– 2 –
pyrimidinyl］– amino］phenyl］benzamide mesylate］。化学结构式为：

HN

甲磺酸伊马替尼是一种白色至类白色至棕褐色或淡黄色结晶粉末，易溶于水，溶于
pH≤5.5 缓冲液，但极微溶至不溶于中性/碱性水缓冲液；不溶于正辛醇、丙酮和乙腈。甲
磺酸伊马替尼有两种晶型，分别为 α 晶型和 β 晶型。

甲磺酸伊马替尼的制备方法很多，按不同原料及路线划分不下十几种。本实验以 2 –
［N –（2 – 甲基 – 5 – 硝基苯基）氨基］– 4 –（3 – 吡啶基）嘧啶（14 – 1）为原料，经氯化
亚锡还原得到 2 –［N –（2 – 甲基 – 5 – 氨基苯基）氨基］– 4 –（3 – 吡啶基）嘧啶（14 – 2），
（14 – 2）直接与 4 –［（4 – 甲基哌嗪基）甲基］苯甲酸缩合得到伊马替尼，再与甲磺酸成盐
得到甲磺酸伊马替尼。

（14-1）

$$\xrightarrow[\text{EA/EtOH}]{\text{SnCl}_2\cdot 2\text{H}_2\text{O}}$$

（14-2）

$$\xrightarrow{\text{HOBt/DMAP/EDCl/DCM/DMF}}$$

伊马替尼

$$\xrightarrow[\text{Isopropanol}]{\text{H}_3\text{C-S-OH}}$$

，$\text{H}_3\text{C-S-OH}$

甲磺酸伊马替尼

【实验预习】

1. 甲磺酸伊马替尼的合成路线有哪些？并对其优缺点进行评价。

2. 还原硝基化合物的常用方法有哪些？羧酸与胺的制备酰胺的方法有哪些？

3. 如何鉴定药物晶型，有哪些方法？

【知识点】

仪器装置，投料过程，还原反应，缩合反应，酸碱调节，萃取，多晶型现象。

【实验步骤】

（一） 2-［N-（2-甲基-5-氨基苯基）氨基］-4-（3-吡啶基）嘧啶（14-2）的制备

1. 原料规格及配比　见表14-1。

表14-1　原料规格及配比表

原料名称	规格	用量	摩尔数	摩尔比
2-［N-甲基-5-硝基苯基）氨基］-4-（3-吡啶基）嘧啶（14-1）	CP	2.0g	0.0065	1
二水氯化亚锡	CP	7.3g	0.0325	5
乙酸乙酯	CP	110ml		
乙醇	CP	5ml		
2mol/L NaOH	CP	50ml		

2. 实验操作　在装有搅拌器、回流冷凝管、温度计的250ml四颈瓶（附注1）中，加入2-［N-甲基-5-硝基苯基）氨基］-4-（3-吡啶基）嘧啶（14-1）2.0g、溶有二水氯化亚锡7.3g的乙酸乙酯和乙醇（10∶1，v/v）的混合溶液55ml，快速搅拌并加热至回流。回流2小时后，冷至室温，用2mol/L NaOH溶液调节溶液pH至9～10，约需50ml（附

注2）。反应液抽滤，滤饼用乙酸乙酯冲洗（20ml×3）（附注3）。收集滤液，分离得到有机相，有机相依次用水50ml、饱和氯化钠溶液50ml洗涤，无水硫酸钠干燥，蒸去乙酸乙酯，得黄色固体1.6g，mp.140～143℃，收率88.89%。

3. 附注

（1）本反应为无水反应，所有仪器均需事先干燥。

（2）可适当提高NaOH溶液的浓度，减少NaOH溶液的用量。

（3）滤饼中含有大量的重金属锡离子，对环境有污染，滤饼集中收集，不可随意丢弃。

4. 思考题

（1）用氯化亚锡还原硝基的反应机制是什么？是否还可以用其他还原剂代替氯化亚锡？

（2）在本反应中，乙醇所起的主要作用是什么？

（二）伊马替尼的制备

1. 原料规格及配比　见表14－2。

表14－2　原料规格及配比表

原料名称	规格	用量	摩尔数	摩尔比
2－[N－（2－甲基－5－氨基苯基）氨基]－4－（3－吡啶基）嘧啶（14－2）	上步反应制得	1.66g	0.006	1
4－[（4－甲基哌嗪基）甲基]苯甲酸二盐酸盐	CP	2.3g	0.0075	1.25
1－羟基苯并三氮唑（HOBt）	CP	1.14g	0.0075	1.25
4－二甲氨基吡啶（DMAP）	CP	0.09g	0.0007	0.125
1－乙基－（3－二甲基氨基丙基）碳酰二亚胺盐酸盐（EDCl）	CP	1.43g	0.0075	1.25
二氯甲烷（DCM）	CP	60ml		
三乙胺（TEA）		2.5ml		
二甲基甲酰胺（DMF）		21ml		

2. 实验操作　在装有搅拌器、温度计、回流冷凝管和恒压滴液漏斗的四颈瓶中，依次加入2－[N－（2－甲基－5－氨基苯基）氨基]－4－（3－吡啶基）嘧啶（14－2）1.66g、4－[（4－甲基哌嗪基）甲基]苯甲酸二盐酸盐2.3g、1－羟基苯并三氮唑（HOBt）1.14g、4－二甲氨基吡啶（DMAP）0.09g、三乙胺（TEA）2.5ml和二甲基甲酰胺（DMF）21ml（附注1）。搅拌，将悬浮液加热到60℃。将1－乙基－（3－二甲基氨基丙基）碳酰二亚胺盐酸盐（EDCl）1.43g溶于二氯甲烷20ml中，并通过恒压滴液漏斗在30分钟内缓慢滴加到反应液中。60℃搅拌反应2小时后，冷至室温继续搅拌1小时。加入二氯甲烷40ml和水20ml，滴加2mol/L氢氧化钠溶液4ml。分离出有机相，依次用水20ml×2、饱和氯化钠溶液20ml×2洗（附注2），无水硫酸钠干燥，蒸除溶剂，得淡棕色固体。在反应瓶内加入磁力搅拌子、异丙醇20ml，在50℃充分搅拌10分钟，抽滤，滤饼用少量异丙醇13.5ml×2洗涤两次，干燥得白色固体2.6g，mp.224.0～226.9℃，收率87.83%。

3. 附注

（1）反应试剂较多，注意加料准确。

（2）有机相用水萃取2～3次，尽可能地除去与二氯甲烷互溶的DMF。

4. 思考题

（1）该反应中的1－羟基苯并三氮唑（HOBt）的作用是什么？是否可用其他试剂代替？

（2）常用的由羧酸与胺制备酰胺的缩合剂有哪些？各有什么特点？

（3）反应操作步骤中，利用异丙醇洗涤的作用是什么？

（三）甲磺酸伊马替尼的制备

1. 原料规格及配比　见表14－3。

表14－3　原料规格及配比表

原料名称	规格	用量	摩尔数	摩尔比
伊马替尼	上步反应制得	2.0g	0.004	1
甲磺酸	CP	0.38g	0.004	1
异丙醇	CP			

2. 实验操作　将伊马替尼2.0g悬浮于异丙醇30ml中，加热到70℃，搅拌10分钟，将溶有甲磺酸0.38g的异丙醇10ml溶液缓慢滴加到伊马替尼异丙醇溶液中，控制时间在15～20分钟滴完。滴加完成后，加热回流30分钟。然后蒸出部分溶剂，剩余物在室温下搅拌结晶（附注1），抽滤，滤饼用少量异丙醇洗涤，干燥后得白色粉末（附注2），mp. 214.0～224.9℃，称重，计算收率。

3. 附注

（1）甲磺酸伊马替尼具有多晶型现象，其中 α 和 β 两种晶型主要用于临床治疗，α 晶型为针状结晶，具有吸湿性、流动性差以及热稳定性差的特点。β 晶型由原研公司诺华开发，受到专利保护，在140℃以下则表现出良好的热稳定性，同时不易吸潮，且流动性较好。本实验得到 α 晶型。

（2）α 晶型中的残留溶剂偏高，这可能与甲磺酸伊马替尼的本身结构有关，分子中含有多个 N，在成盐结晶过程中会与溶剂发生分子间的缔合作用。

4. 思考题

（1）为什么要控制滴加甲磺酸异丙醇溶液的速度？

（2）如何除去甲磺酸伊马替尼中的残留溶剂？

（3）同一种药物，不同晶型之间会存在哪些性质上的差异？

【伊马替尼的结构表征】

熔点：224.0～226.9℃。

^{1}H－NMR：结构正确（附图14－1）。

HRMS（ESI$^+$）：494.26629 [M＋H]$^+$（附图14－2）。

EI－MS（m/z）：494 [M＋H]$^+$。

HPLC 纯度：99.9%。

HPLC 测试的色谱条件：

色谱柱：十八烷基硅烷键合硅胶（4.6mm×250mm，5μm）。

流速：1.0ml/min。

进样量：10μl。

检测波长：267nm。

流动相 A：辛烷磺酸钠溶液－甲醇（65：35）。使用前需超声脱气。

流动相 B：辛烷磺酸钠溶液－甲醇（45：55）。使用前需超声脱气。

按表 14 - 4 进行线性梯度洗脱。

表 14 - 4　洗脱流程

时间/min	流动相 A/%	流动相 B/%
0	75	25
15	75	25
20	25	75
25	0	100
30	0	100

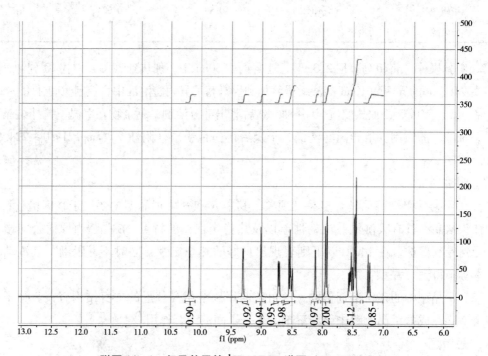

附图 14 - 1　伊马替尼的 ^{1}H - NMR 谱图（DMSO - d$_{6}$）

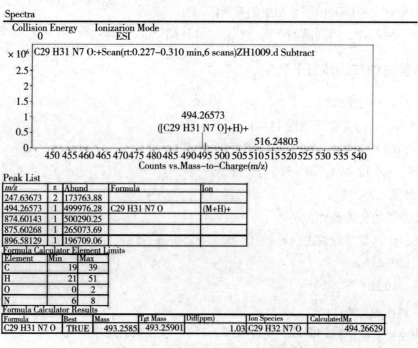

附图 14 - 2　伊马替尼的 HRMS 谱图（ESI^{+}）

Experiment 14　Synthesis of Imatinib Mesylate

Experimental aim

1. Learn the synthesis process and clinical use of imatinib.

2. Understand the effect of crystalline form on drug properties.

3. Train the basic principles and operations of condensation and reduction reactions.

4. Practice the method for crystallization and extraction.

Experimental principles

Imatinib mesylate

$4 - [(4 - methyl - 1 - piperazinyl) methyl] - N - [4 - methyl - 3 -$
$[[4 - (3 - pyridinyl) - 2 - pyrimidinyl] - amino] phenyl] benzamide mesylate$

　Imatinib mesylate is a white to off – white to brownish or yellowish tinged crystalline powder. It is very soluble in water and soluble in aqueous buffers $pH \leqslant 5.5$ but is very slightly soluble to insoluble in neutral/alkaline aqueous buffers. It is insoluble in n – octanol, acetone and acetonitrile. There are two crystal forms of imatinib mesylate, α and β.

　There are more than ten preparation methods of imatinib in literature, according to the starting materials and synthetic processes. In this experiment, $2 - [N - (2 - methyl - 5 - nitrophenyl)$ amino $] - 4 - (3 - pyridinyl) pyrimidine (14 - 1)$ is used as starting material and it is reduced with stannous chloride to $2 - [N - (2 - methyl - 5 - aminophenyl) amino] - 4 - (3 - pyridyl) pyrimidine$ $(14 - 2)$. $(14 - 2)$ was directly condensed with $4 - [(4 - methylpiperazinyl) methyl] benzoic acid$ to obtain imatinib, and then imatinib is salted with methanesulfonic acid to obtain imatinib mesylate.

（14–1）　　　$\xrightarrow[\text{EA/EtOH}]{\text{SnCl}_2 \cdot 2\text{H}_2\text{O}}$　　　（14–2）

$\xrightarrow{\text{HOBt/DMAP/EDCl/DCM/DMF}}$

Imatine

$$H_3C-\overset{\overset{\displaystyle O}{\|}}{\underset{\underset{\displaystyle O}{\|}}{S}}-OH \xrightarrow{\text{Isopropanol}}$$

Imatinib mesylate

Pre - lab preparation

1. Review the all synthesis methods of imatinib and evaluate their advantages and disadvantages.

2. Summarize the reduction methods of nitro group to amino group. Review the methods for the preparation of amide by acylation between carboxylic acid and amine.

3. Learn the methods to identify the crystal forms.

Knowledge point

Set – up of reaction apparatus, adding procedures of chemical reagents, condensation reaction, reduction reaction, acid – base adjustment, extraction, polymorphism.

Experiment procedures

I. Synthesis of 2 – [N – (2 – methyl – 5 – aminophenyl) amino] – 4 – (3 – pyridyl) pyrimidine(14 – 2)

1. Materials(Table 14 – 1)

Table 14 – 1　Specification and ratio of raw materials

Materials	Specifications	Amount	Mol	Mol ratio
2 – [N – (2 – methyl – 5 – nitrophenyl) amino] – 4 – (3 – pyridinyl) pyrimidine (14 – 1)	CP	2.0g	0.0065	1
$SnCl_2 \cdot 2H_2O$	CP	7.3g	0.0325	5
Ethyl acetate	CP	110ml		
Ethanol	CP	5ml		
2mol/L NaOH	CP	50ml		

2. Procedures　To a 250ml four neck flask equipped with stirrer, condenser and thermometer (Note 1), 2 – [N – (2 – methyl – 5 – nitrophenyl) amino] – 4 – (3 – pyridinyl) pyrimidine(14 – 1) and $SnCl_2 \cdot 2H_2O$ dissolved in a mixture of ethyl acetate and ethanol(55ml, 10 : 1, v/v) were added. The reaction solution was heated to refluxing and kept refluxing for 2h. The solution was cooled to room temperature, and the solution was adjusted to pH 9 ~ 10 with 2mol/L aqueous sodium hydroxide solution(about 50ml) (Note 2). Then the solution was sucking filtrated and the filter cake was washed with ethyl acetate(20ml × 3) (Note 3). The filtrate organic layer was washed in turn with water 50ml and saturated sodium chloride solution 50ml. Then the organic layer was dried over

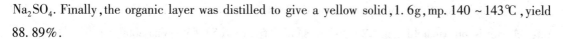

Na_2SO_4. Finally, the organic layer was distilled to give a yellow solid, 1.6g, mp. 140 ~ 143℃, yield 88.89%.

3. Notes

Note 1: All instruments should be dried before use.

Note 2: The concentration of NaOH solution can be appropriately increased to reduce the amount of NaOH solution.

Note 3: The Sn^{2+} was oxidized to Sn^{4+} in this reaction, which presented in the filter cake and could cause environmental pollution. The filter cake should be collected carefully and is not throwed away after the experiment.

4. Questions

(1) Give an explanation for the mechanism of the reduction reaction, and could $SnCl_2 \cdot 2H_2O$ be substituted by other reagent in this reaction?

(2) What is the effect of ethanol?

Ⅱ. Synthesis of Imatinib

1. Materials(Table 14 – 2)

Table 14 – 2   Specification and ratio of raw materials

Materials	Specifications	Amount	Mol	Mol ratio
2 – [N – (2 – methyl – 5 – aminophenyl) amino] – 4 – (3 – pyridyl) pyrimidine(14 – 2)	Prepared in last step	1.66g	0.006	1
4 – (4 – methyl – piperazinomethyl) benzoic aciddihydrochloride	CP	2.3g	0.0075	1.25
1 – hydroxybenzotriazole(HOBt)	CP	1.14g	0.0075	1.25
4 – dimethylaminopyridine(DMAP)	CP	0.09g	0.0007	0.125
1 – ethyl – (3 – dimethylaminopropyl) carbamide hydrochloride(EDCl)	CP	1.43g	0.0075	1.25
Dichloromethane(DCM)	CP	60ml		
Triethylamine(TEA)		2.5ml		
Dimethylformamide(DMF)		21ml		

2. Procedures   In a four – necked flask equipped with agitator, thermometer, reflux condenser and constant pressure drop funnel were added 2 – [N – (2 – methyl – 5 – aminophenyl) amino] – 4 – (3 – pyridyl) pyrimidine (14 – 2) 1.66g, 4 – (4 – methyl – piperazinomethyl) benzoic acid dihydrochloride 2.3g, HOBT 1.14g, DMAP 0.09g, TEA 2.5ml and DMF 21ml (Note 1). The suspension was stirred and heated to 60℃ and a solution of EDCl 1.43g in dichloromethane 20ml was slowly added through a constant pressure drop funnel during 30 minutes. The reaction solution was stirred at 60℃ for 2 hours. The reaction mixture was cooled to room temperature and stirred at rt for 1 hour and then dichloromethane 40ml and water 20ml were added and 2mol/L NaOH solution 4ml was added dropwise. The organic phase was separated and washed twice with water 20ml × 2 and saturated sodium chloride solution 20ml × 2 (Note 2). The organic layer was dried over Na_2SO_4 and was distilled to give a brownish solid. The humid solid was added isopropnol 20ml and a magnetic bar, the solution was stirred for 10mins at 50℃. Then the solution was filtered and the filter cake was washed with isopropanol 13. 5ml ×2. A white solid 2. 6g, yield 87. 83% was obtained.

3. Notes

Note 1: There are many reaction agents, please pay attention to accurate amounts.

Note 2: During extraction, the organic phase should be extracted 2 ~ 3 times with water to remove DMF which is miscible with dichloromethane as much as possible.

4. Question

(1) What is the role of 1 – hydroxybenzotriazole (HOBt) in this reaction and could it be substituted by other reagent?

(2) What are the commonly used condensationreagents for preparation amide from carboxylic acid and amine? How about their characteristics of these reagents?

(3) In the reaction procedure, what is the role of isopropanol?

Ⅲ. Systhesis of Imatinib mesylate

1. Materials (Table 14 – 3)

Table 14 – 3　Specification and ratio of raw materials

Materials	Specifications	Amount	Mol	Mol ratio
Imatinib	Prepared in last step	2. 0g	0. 004	1
Methanesulfonic acid	CP	0. 38g	0. 004	1
Isopropanol	CP			

2. Procedures　Imatinib 2. 0g was suspended in isopropanol 30ml and heated at 70℃ for 10min. To the mixtures of imatinib and isopropyl alcohol solution, methanesulfonic acid 0. 38g in isopropanol 10ml wad added dropwise slowly during 15 to 20 minutes. Then the mixture was heat to refluxing for 30 minutes and half parts of isopropanol in the mixture was distillated out. The residue was stirred for crystallization at room temperature (Note 1). The crystal was collected by sucting filtration and washed with isopropanol. A white solid was obtained, mp. 214. 0 ~ 224. 9℃ (Note 2), weight and for calculating yield.

3. Notes

Note 1: Imatinib mesylate has polycrystalline form, of which α and β are mainly used in clinical. α crystal is needle crystal with hygroscopicity, poor fluidity and poor thermal stability. β crystal, a original developed form by Novartis, is protected by patent. Under 140℃, it shows good thermal stability, is not easy to absorb moisture, and has good fluidity. In this experiment, α crystal form was obtained.

Note 2: The α crystal form contains higher residual solvent, which may be related to the structure of imatinib mesylate. There are many nitrogen atoms in the molecule, which will associate with the solvent in the process of salt formation and crystallization.

4. Questions

(1) The addition ration of methanesulfonic acid in isopropyl alcohol to the mixtures of imatinib and isopropyl alcohol solution should be controlled, and give an explanation.

(2) How to remove the residual solvent inimatinib mesylate in this experiment?

（3）What are the properties of different crystal types of the same drug?

【Characterization of Imatinib mesylate】

Melting point：224. 0 ~ 226. 9℃.

$^1H - NMR$：Conforms（Attached figure 14 - 1）.

HRMS（ESI$^+$）：494. 26629（M + H$^+$）（Attached figure 14 - 2）.

EI - MS（m/z）：494[M + H]$^+$.

HPLC：99. 9%.

HPLC conditions：

Column：C18（4. 6mm × 250mm, 5μm）.

Flow rate：1. 0ml/min.

Injection volume：10μl.

Detection wavelength：267nm.

Mobile phase A：Sodium 1 - octanesulfonate - Methanol（65 : 35）.

Mobile phase B：Sodium 1 - octanesulfonate - Methanol（45 : 55）.

Perform gradient elution according to the Table 14 - 4.

Ultrasonic degassing before use.

Table 14 - 4 Flution gradient

Time/min	Mobile phase A/%	Mobile phase B/%
0	75	25
15	75	25
20	25	75
25	0	100
30	0	100

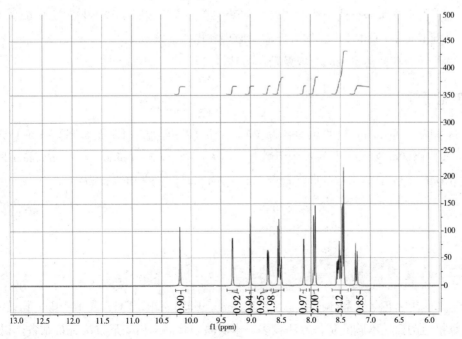

Attached figure 14 -1 $^1H - NMR$ spectrum of imatinib（DMSO - d$_6$）

Spectra

Collision Energy	Ionizarion Mode
0	ESI

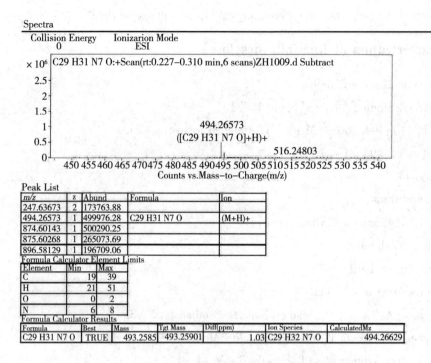

Peak List

m/z	z	Abund	Formula	Ion
247.63673	2	173763.88		
494.26573	1	499976.28	C29 H31 N7 O	(M+H)+
874.60143	1	500290.25		
875.60268	1	265073.69		
896.58129	1	196709.06		

Formula Calculator Element Limits

Element	Min	Max
C	19	39
H	21	51
O	0	2
N	6	8

Formula Calculator Results

Formula	Best	Mass	Tgt Mass	Diff(ppm)	Ion Species	CalculatedMz
C29 H31 N7 O	TRUE	493.2585	493.25901	1.03	C29 H32 N7 O	494.26629

Attached figure 14 – 2　HRMS spectrum of imatinib（ESI⁺）

实验十五　西达本胺的合成

【实验目的】

1. 了解西达本胺的临床用途、作用靶标、工业生产及市场情况。
2. 通过对西达本胺合成路线的比较，使学生掌握选择实际生产工艺的几个基本要求。
3. 掌握 Knoevenagel 反应、缩合反应的原理和操作要求。
4. 学习原料药西达本胺的合成及精制方法。

【实验原理】

西达本胺（chidamide）的化学名为（E）– N –（2 – 氨基 – 4 – 氟苯基）– 4 –（（3 –（吡啶 – 3 – 基）丙烯酰胺基）甲基）苯甲酰胺，[（E）– N –（2 – amino – 4 – fluorophenyl）– 4 –（（3 –（pyridin – 3 – yl）acrylamido）methyl）benzamide]。化学结构式为：

西达本胺为白色针状晶体或结晶性粉末，mp. 200.5 ~ 202.1℃，易溶于酸，微溶于水。

文献报道的西达本胺的制备方法较多，本实验中我们采用如下方法进行制备。以 3 – 吡啶甲醛（15 – 1）为原料，在吡啶和哌啶的作用下与丙二酸（15 – 2）发生 Knoevenagel 反应生成（E）-3-（吡啶-3-基）丙烯酸（15-3），然后与4-氨甲基苯甲酸发生缩合反应制备得到中间体（E）-4-（（3-（吡啶-3-基）丙烯酰氨基）甲基）苯甲酸（15-4）。最后（15-4）再与3,4-二氨基氟苯进行酰胺化反应，得到西达本胺。

（图）

【实验预习】

1. 西达本胺的合成方法有哪些？并对其优缺点进行评价。
2. 常见由羧酸和胺制备酰胺的缩合剂有哪些？
3. Knoevenagel 反应机制是什么？

【知识点】

仪器装置，投料过程，缩合反应，歧化反应，重结晶，纯度测试，TLC 监控。

【实验步骤】

（一）（E）-3-（吡啶-3-基）丙烯酸（15-3）的合成

1. 原料规格及配比　见表 15-1。

表 15-1　原料规格及配比表

原料名称	规格	用量	摩尔数	摩尔比
吡啶甲醛（15-1）	CP	10g	93.4mmol	1
丙二酸（15-2）	AR	9.8g	93.4mmol	1
吡啶	AR	4.48g	56mmol	0.6
哌啶	CP	0.44g	5.6mmol	0.06
1mol/L 盐酸	CP			

　　2. 实验操作　在 100ml 三颈瓶中加入吡啶甲醛（15-1）、丙二酸（15-2）、吡啶和哌啶（附注1），磁力搅拌，升温回流 2 小时后，TLC 监测反应完毕（展开剂 DCM：MeOH = 10：1 + 2 滴 TEA）（附注2），停止反应。浓缩反应液蒸除溶剂，用 1mol/L 盐酸溶液调至 pH=3，抽滤，得白色固体（15-3）。

3. 附注

（1）本反应中吡啶既作为溶剂，同时又作为催化反应进行的碱，反应过程中应当注意避免原料吡啶甲醛发生歧化反应。

（2）DCM 为二氯甲烷，TEA 为三乙胺。

（二）（E）-4-（（3-（吡啶-3-基）丙烯酰氨基）甲基）苯甲酸（15-4）的制备

1. 原料规格及配比　见表 15-2。

表 15-2　原料规格及配比表

原料名称	规格	用量	摩尔数	摩尔比
（E）-3-（吡啶-3-基）丙烯酸（15-3）	上步反应制得	5.0g	33.5mmol	1
N，N'-羰基二咪唑	AR	5.5g	33.5mmol	1
无水四氢呋喃	AR	100ml		
对氨甲基苯甲酸	AR	5.0g	33.5mmol	1
氢氧化钠	AR	1.35g	33.5mmol	1

2. 实验操作　在 100ml 三颈瓶中，加入 N，N'-羰基二咪唑 5.5g（附注 1）和无水四氢呋喃 50ml（附注 2），搅拌形成混悬液，然后滴加（E）-3-（吡啶-3-基）丙烯酸（15-3）5.0g，搅拌，加热至 65℃反应 2 小时，反应液变澄清，TLC（展开剂 DCM：MeOH=20：1）监测原料 3-（吡啶-3-基）丙烯酸（15-3）完全转化为中间体，备用。

另取 200ml 三颈瓶，加入对氨甲基苯甲酸 5.0g、氢氧化钠 1.35g 和无水四氢呋喃 50ml，搅拌加热至 65℃后，滴加上述备用的中间体溶液，30 分钟加完，然后室温反应 2 小时，TLC（展开剂 DCM：MeOH=20：1~7：1）监测反应完毕后，停止反应。旋转蒸发器上真空蒸除溶剂，用 1mol/L 盐酸溶液调至 pH=5，冰浴冷却得大量固体，抽滤，滤饼用少量冰水淋洗得白色固体。

3. 附注

（1）CDI 的用量如果过多会生成大量的脲类副产物。

（2）溶剂无水四氢呋喃要预先干燥。

（三）西达本胺的制备

1. 原料规格及配比　见表 15-3。

表 15-3　原料规格及配比表

原料名称	规格	用量	摩尔数	摩尔比
（E）-4-（（3-（吡啶-3-基）丙烯酰氨基）甲基）苯甲酸（15-4）	上步反应制得	5.0g	17.8mmol	1
N，N'-羰基二咪唑	AR	2.9g	17.8mmol	1
无水四氢呋喃	AR	100ml		
4-氟-1，2-苯二胺	AR	2.8g	22.2mmol	1.2
三氟乙酸	AR	2.0g	17.8mmol	1

2. 实验操作 于 100ml 三颈瓶中加入 N，N' – 碳酰二咪唑 2.9g、(E) – 4 – （（3 – （吡啶 – 3 – 基）丙烯酰氨基）甲基）苯甲酸（15 – 4）5.0g 以及无水四氢呋喃 50ml，45℃ 搅拌反应 1 小时。反应结束后，冷却至室温。加入到另一溶有 4 – 氟 – 1，2 – 苯二胺 2.8g 和三氟乙酸 2.0g 的四氢呋喃 50ml 溶液的 200ml 三颈瓶中，室温搅拌反应 3 小时。析出固体，抽滤，四氢呋喃洗涤，干燥得西达本胺粗品，再经乙醇重结晶、干燥得白色固体。

3. 思考题

（1）3 – 吡啶甲醛在碱性条件下会发生什么副反应？生成何种副产物？

（2）在西达本胺的合成中，为何主要是 3，4 – 二氨基氟苯中 4 位的氨基与 (E) – 4 – （（3 – （吡啶 – 3 – 基）丙烯酰氨基）甲基）苯甲酸（15 – 4）进行缩合而不是 3 位氨基，请从反应机制进行解释。

【西达本胺的结构表征】

熔点：200.5 ~ 201.1℃。

^1H – NMR：结构正确（附图 15 – 1）。

HRMS（ESI^+）：391.1569（$M + H^+$）（附图 15 – 2）。

HPLC 纯度：98.5%。

HPLC 测试的色谱条件：

色谱柱：Venusil MP – C18（4.6mm × 250mm，5μm）。

流速：1ml/min。

检测波长：254nm。

柱温：25℃。

流动相：0.1% 醋酸溶液 – 乙腈梯度洗脱，乙腈 25% ~ 60%（13 分钟）、60% ~ 25%（3 分钟）、25%（4 分钟）。使用前需超声脱气。

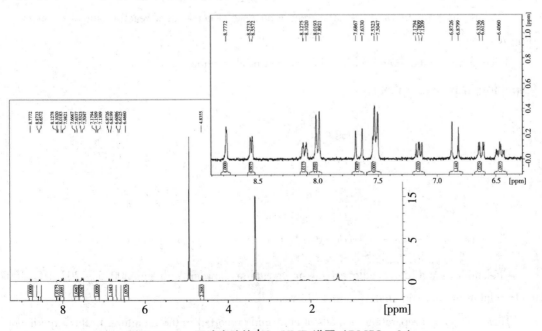

附图 15 – 1 西达本胺的 ^1H – NMR 谱图（DMSO – d_6）

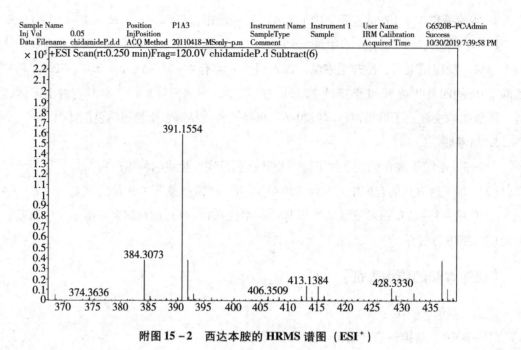

Sample Name		Position	P1A3		Instrument Name	Instrument 1	User Name	G6520B–PC\Admin
Inj Vol	0.05	InjPosition			SampleType	Sample	IRM Calibration	Success
Data Filename	chidamideP.d.d	ACQ Method	20110418–MSonly–p.m		Comment		Acquired Time	10/30/2019 7:39:58 PM

×10⁵ +ESI Scan(rt:0.250 min)Frag=120.0V chidamideP.d Subtract(6)

附图 15 – 2　西达本胺的 HRMS 谱图（ESI⁺）

Experiment 15　Synthesis of Chidamide

Experimental aim

1. Get preliminary knowledge of the clinical use, action mechanism, industrial manufacture and market conditions of chidamide.

2. Learn how to selecta practical process according to comparison of several different synthetic routes.

3. Learn the principle and operation requirements of Knoevenagel reaction and the condens – ation reaction.

4. Train the synthetic and purification method of chidamide.

Experimental principles

Chidamide

$(E) - N - (2 - amino - 4 - fluorophenyl) - 4 - ((3 - (pyridin - 3 - yl) acrylamido) methyl) benzamide$

Chidamide is a white needle crystal or crystalline powder with mp. 200. 5 ~ 202. 1℃. It is freely soluble in acid and slightly soluble in water.

There are many preparation methods of chidamide reported in the literature. In this experiment, we use the following method to prepare it. Nicotinaldehyde(15 – 1) was used as raw material to react with malonic acid(15 − 2) in the presence of pyridine and piperidine through Knoevenagel reaction to form (*E*) − 3 − (pyridin − 3 − yl) acrylic acid (15 − 3) , and then reacts with 4 − aminomethylbenzoic acid to produce(*E*) − 4 − ((3 − (pyridin − 3 − yl) acrylamido) methyl) benzoic acid(15 − 4). Finally , (15 − 4) reacts with 3 , 4 − diaminofluorobenzene by amide reaction to give chidamide.

Chidamide

Experimental preparation

1. Summarize the all synthesis methods of chidamide and give an evaluation of their advantages and disadvantages.

2. What are the commonly condensing agents for the preparation of amides from carboxylic acids and amines?

3. What is the reaction mechanism for Knoevenagel reaction?

Knowledge point

Set − up of reaction apparatus , adding procedures of chemical reagents , condensation reaction , disproportionation , recrystallization , purity test , TLC operation.

Experiment procedures

I. Synthesis of (*E*) − 3 − (pyridin − 3 − yl) acrylic acid(15 − 3)

1. Materials(Table 15 − 1)

Table 15 − 1   Specification and ratio of raw materials

Materials	Specification	Amount	Mol	Mol ratio
Nicotinaldehyde(15 − 1)	CP	10g	93. 4mmol	1
Malonic acid(15 − 2)	AR	9. 8g	93. 4mmol	1
Pyridine	AR	4. 48g	56mmol	0. 6
Piperidine	CP	0. 44g	5. 6mmol	0. 06
1mol/L hydrochloric acid	CP			

2. Procedures   In a 100ml three neck flask, nicotinaldehyde(15 – 1)10g, malonic acid(15 – 2)9. 8g, pyridine 4. 48g and piperidine 0. 44g were added(Note 1). The mixture was stirred with a magnetical bar, and heated to reflux for 2h. The end point of the reaction was monitored by TLC (DCM : MeOH = 10 : 1 + 2 drop STEA)(Note 2). The mixture was concentrated to remove the solvent, and the residual was adjusted to pH = 3 with 1mol/L hydrochloric acid. (E) – 3 – (pyridin – 3 – yl)acrylic acid(15 – 3)as a white solid was obtained after filtration.

3. Notes

Note 1: In this reaction, pyridine acts both as a solvent and a base for the catalytic reaction. During the reaction, it should be paied more attention to avoid disproportionation reaction of the nicotinaldehyde.

Note 2: DCM is dichloromethane; TEA is triethyl amine.

Ⅱ. Synthesis of (E) – 4 – ((3 – (pyridin – 3 – yl)acrylamido)methyl)benzoic acid(15 – 4)

1. Materials(Table 15 – 2)

Table 15 – 2   Specification and ratio of raw materials

Materials	Specification	Amount	Mol	Mol ratio
(E) – 3 – (pyridin – 3 – yl)acrylic acid(15 – 3)	Prepared in last step	5. 0g	33. 5mmol	1
N,N' – carbonyldiimidazole	AR	5. 5g	33. 5mmol	1
Anhydrous tetrahydrofuran	AR	100ml		
4 – aminomethylbenzoic acid	AR	5. 0g	33. 5mmol	1
Sodium hydroxide	AR	1. 35g	33. 5mmol	1

2. Procedures   In a 100ml three neck flask, N,N' – carbonyldiimidazole 5. 5g(Note 1) and anhydrous tetrahydrofuran 50ml(Note 2) were added. A suspension formed and was stirred. To the suspension, (E) – 3 – (pyridin – 3 – yl)acrylic acid(15 – 3) was added dropwise. The reaction solution was stirred at 65℃ for 2h. The reaction solution became clear, and TLC was used to monitor the complete conversion of(15 – 3)into an intermediate(DCM : MeOH = 20 : 1).

In a 200ml three neck flask, aminomethylbenzoic acid 5. 0g, sodium hydroxide 1. 35g and anhydrous tetrahydrofuran 50ml were added. The solution was stirred and heated to 65℃, and the intermediate was added dropwise to the solution during 30min. The reaction was stirred for 2h at room temperature. The end point of the reaction was monitored by TLC(DCM : MeOH = 20 : 1 ~ 7 : 1). The mixture was evaporated to dryness and the residual was adjusted to pH = 5 with a 1mol/L hydrochloric acid and was cooled in ice bath. A white solid deposited was collected by filtration, washed with ice – water.

3. Notes

Note 1: If the amount of CDI is too large, a large amount of urea – containing by – products will be formed.

Note 2: The tetrahydrofuran should be dried before using.

Ⅲ. Synthesis of Chidamide

1. Materials(Table 15 −3)

Table 15 −3 　Specification and ratio of raw materials

Materials	Specification	Amount	Mol	Mol ratio
(E) − 4 − ((3 − (pyridin − 3 − yl) acrylamido) methyl) benzoic acid(15 −4)	Prepared in last step	5. 0g	17. 8mmol	1
N,N' − carbonyldiimidazole	AR	2. 9g	17. 8mmol	1
Anhydrous tetrahydrofuran	AR	100ml		
4 − fluoro − 1,2 − phenyldiamine	AR	2. 8g	22. 2mmol	1. 2
Trifluoroacetic acid	AR	2. 0g	17. 8mmol	1

2. Procedures　In a 100ml three neck flask, N,N' − carbonyldiimidazole 2. 9g, (E) − 4 − ((3 − (pyridin − 3 − yl) acrylamido) methyl) benzoic acid (15 − 4) 5. 0g and anhydrous tetrahydrofuran 50ml was added. The mixture was stirred at 45℃ for 1h. After cooling to room temperature, the reaction mixture was added to another solution of 4 − fluoro − 1,2 − phenyldiamine 2. 8g and in trifluoroacetic acid 2. 0g in tetrahydrofuran 50ml in a 200ml three neck flask at room temperature. The solution was stirred for 3 hours at room temperature. A white solid deposited and was collected by filtration, washed with tetrahydrofuran and then dried to give chidamide crude, recrystallized from ethanol and dried to a white solid.

3. Questions

(1)What side reactions will take place for nicotinaldehyde under alkaline conditions? What kind of by − products are generated?

(2)In the synthesis of chidamide, why will(E) − 4 − ((3 − (pyridin − 3 − yl) acrylamido) methyl) benzoic acid(15 −4) only react with the 4 − amino group rather than the 3 − amino group? Please give its reaction mechanism.

【Characterization of Chidamide】

Melting point:200. 5 ~201. 1℃.

^{1}H − NMR:Conforms(Attached figure 15 − 1).

HRMS(ESI $^+$):391. 1569(M + H $^+$)(Attached figure 15 −2).

HPLC purity:98. 5%

HPLC conditions:

Column:Venusil MP − C18(4. 6mm × 250mm,5μm).

Flow rate:1ml/min.

Detection wavelength:254nm.

Column temperature:25℃.

Mobile phase:0. 1% acetic acid solution − acetonitrile gradient elution, acetonitrile 25% ~ 60%(13min),60% ~25%(3min),25%(4min).

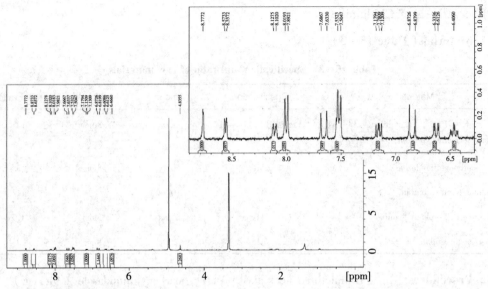

Attached figure 15 – 1 ^{1}H – NMR spectrum of chidamide（300 MHz，DMSO – d$_6$）

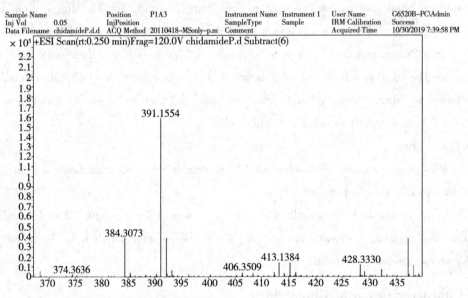

Attached figure 15 – 2   HRMS spectrum of chidamide（ESI$^+$）

实验十六   阿昔洛韦的合成

【实验目的】

1. 了解阿昔洛韦的临床用途、工业生产及市场情况。
2. 掌握阿昔洛韦的合成方法。
3. 掌握减压蒸馏的基本原理和操作。

【实验原理】

阿昔洛韦（acyclovir）的化学名为9 – （2 – 羟乙氧基甲基）鸟嘌呤，[9 – （2 – hydroxyethoxymethyl） guanine]。化学结构式为：

阿昔洛韦为白色结晶性粉末，无臭，无味，mp. 256～257℃，易溶于氢氧化钠溶液，略溶于冰醋酸或热水，在乙醚或二氯甲烷中几乎不溶。

阿昔洛韦的工业生产以下述路线为主。以鸟嘌呤（16－1）为原料，乙酰化得 N, N－二乙酰鸟嘌呤（DAG）（16－2），再与（2－乙酰氧基乙氧基）甲基乙酸酯反应得二乙酰基阿昔洛韦（DACV）（16－3），最后经碱水解得阿昔洛韦（ACV）。

【实验预习】

1. 阿昔洛韦的合成方法有哪些？并对其优缺点进行评价。
2. 总结减压蒸馏的基本操作、注意事项。
3. 热过滤的目的是什么？具体的步骤包括哪些？

【知识点】

仪器装置，投料过程，酰化反应，减压蒸馏，热过滤，酸碱调节，纯度检查。

【实验步骤】

（一）N, N－二乙酰鸟嘌呤（DAG）（16－2）的合成

1. 原料规格及配比　见表16－1。

表16－1　原料规格及配比表

原料名称	规格	用量	摩尔数	摩尔比
鸟嘌呤（16－1）	工业品	5.0g	0.03	1
醋酐	AR	32ml	0.33	11
冰乙酸	CP	16ml		
NaHSO$_4$	CP	0.12g	0.001	0.033
乙醇	CP			

2. 实验操作   在250ml 单口烧瓶中，依次加入鸟嘌呤5.0g（0.03mol）、NaHSO₄ 0.12g（1mmol）、醋酐32ml 和冰乙酸16ml，130℃加热回流12小时，反应结束后，减压蒸馏除去部分溶剂（附注），剩余物抽滤，滤饼依次用乙醇和水洗涤，放入烘箱中80℃烘干，得淡黄色粉末状固体4.6g，收率65.3%。

3. 附注   在进行减压蒸馏除去溶剂时，应蒸除体系内2/3溶剂，冷却析晶后，过滤获得产品。

4. 思考题

（1）开始减压蒸馏时，为什么要先抽气再加热？而结束时为什么要先移开热源，再停止抽气？

（2）回流温度过高会对反应体系有何影响？

（二）二乙酰基阿昔洛韦（DACV）（16-3）的合成

1. 原料规格及配比   见表16-2。

表16-2   原料规格及配比表

原料名称	规格	用量	摩尔数	摩尔比
N，N-二乙酰鸟嘌呤（DAG）（16-2）	上步自制	4.6g	0.019	1
（2-乙酰氧基乙氧基）甲基乙酸酯	CP	7.49g	0.043	2.24
NaHSO₄	CP	0.25g	0.002	0.1
甲苯	CP	30ml		

2. 实验操作   在250ml 三口烧瓶中加入N，N-二乙酰鸟嘌呤（DAG）（16-2）4.6g（0.019mol）、NaHSO₄ 0.25g、甲苯30ml（附注1），搅拌。加热至回流分水（附注2），待分水完毕后，开始滴加（2-乙酰氧基乙氧基）甲基乙酸酯7.49g（附注3），滴加完毕后，回流反应10小时。停止加热、冷却、抽滤、滤饼用水洗涤、压紧抽干后，放入烘箱烘干，得淡黄色粉末状固体二乙酰基阿昔洛韦（DACV）（16-3）4.3g，收率71.7%。

3. 附注

（1）N，N-二乙酰鸟嘌呤（DAG）的嘌呤环上7位的N 和9位的N 都可与（2-乙酰氧基乙氧基）甲基乙酸酯发生如下反应，用甲苯作溶剂可减少副产物的发生。

（2）采用分水器，经气化的过量甲苯直接流入反应体系中，逸出的未反应甲苯蒸气和水蒸气经冷凝后进入分水器，将上层未反应的甲苯干燥后，继续气化进入反应体系。

（3）此反应为密闭体系，采用恒压滴液漏斗防止溶剂的挥发。

4. 思考题

（1）分水器如何使用，注意事项有哪些？

（2）简述该步合成的反应机制。

（三）阿昔洛韦的制备

1. 原料规格及配比 见表16-3。

表16-3 原料规格及配比表

原料名称	规格	用量	摩尔数	摩尔比
二乙酰基阿昔洛韦（DACV）（16-3）	上步自制	4.3g	0.014	1
Na_2CO_3	AR	1.4g	0.13	10
水		30ml		
18mol/L 盐酸	自制			

2. 实验操作 在250ml 三口烧瓶中，加入二乙酰基阿昔洛韦（DACV）（16-3）4.3g、Na_2CO_3 1.4g、H_2O 30ml，加热回流2小时，趁热过滤（附注1），滤液用18mol/L 盐酸调pH 至7（附注2），有大量白色固体生成，过滤，水洗，烘干。最终得白色粉状固体2.11g，收率69.2%。

3. 附注

（1）产品溶解度随温度变化，温度升高，溶解度增大。采用趁热过滤，将产物保留在滤液中，从而达到与杂质分离的目的。

（2）用盐酸调节生成氯化钠盐，后处理简单。为避免产品的损失，调节过程中要缓慢滴加调节至中性。

4. 思考题 从此反应来看，说出其他的水解原料，并解释原因。

【阿昔洛韦的结构表征】

熔点：255.5~257℃。

^1H-NMR：结构正确（附图16-1）。

HRMS（ESI^+）：226.11（$M+H^+$）（附图16-2）。

HPLC 纯度：99.9%。

HPLC 测试的色谱条件：

色谱柱：十八烷基硅烷键合硅胶（4.6mm×250mm，5μm）。

检测波长：254nm。

柱温：35℃。

流动相：以水为流动相A，甲醇为流动相B，按表16-4进行梯度洗脱。使用前需超声脱气。

表16-4 梯度洗脱表

时间/min	流动相A/%	流动相B/%
0	94	6
15	94	6
40	65	35
41	94	6
51	94	6

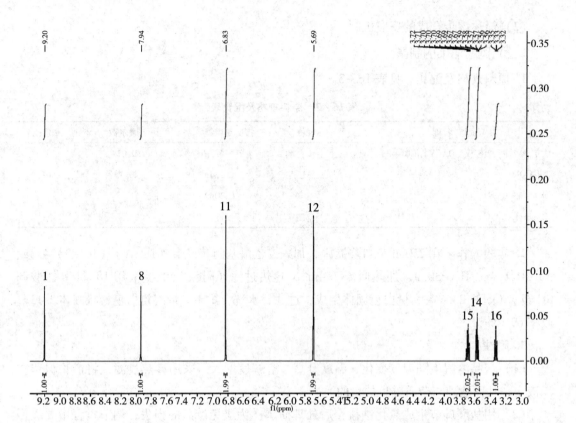

附图 16 – 1　阿昔洛韦的 ^{1}H – NMR 谱图（DMSO – d$_6$）

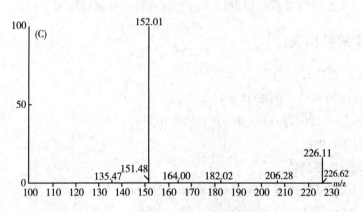

附图 16 – 2　阿昔洛韦的 HRMS 谱图（ESI$^+$）

Experiment 16　　Synthesis of Acyclovir

Experimental aim

1. Understand the clinical use, industrial manufacture process and market conditions of acyclovir。

2. Practice the synthesis method of acyclovir.

3. Train the basic principles and operations of vacuum distillation.

Experimental principles

Acyclovir
9 – (2 – hydroxyethoxymethyl) guanine

Acyclovir is a white crystalline powder, odorless and tasteless with mp. $256 \sim 257°C$. It is freely soluble in sodium hydroxide solution, sparingly soluble in glacial acetic acid or hot water, and practically insoluble in diethyl ether or dichloromethane.

In industrial manufacture process of acyclovir, Guanine (16 – 1) as a starting material reacted with acetic anhydride to give N, N – diacetylguanine (DAG) (16 – 2). Then (16 – 2) reacts with (2 – acetoxyethoxy) methyl acetate to obtain diacetyl acyclovir (DACV) (16 – 3). Acyclovir (ACV) is obtained by alkaline hydrolysis of diacetyl acyclovir (DACV) (16 – 3).

(16-1)   (16-2) DAG   (16-3) DACV   Acyclovir, ACV

Pre – lab preparation

1. Summarize the synthetic methods of acyclovir and evaluate their advantages and disadvantages.

2. Review the operation and precautions for vacuum distillation.

3. Review the purpose of filtration while hot and its specific steps.

Knowledge point

Set – up of reaction apparatus, adding procedures of chemical reagents, acylation reaction, vacuum distillation, filtrating while hot, acid – base adjustment, purity check.

Experiment procedures

Ⅰ. Synthesis of N, N – diacetylguanine (DAG) (16 – 2)

1. Materials (Table 16 – 1)

Table 16 – 1   Specification and ratio of raw materials

Materials	Specifications	Amount	Mol	Mol ratio
Guanine (16 – 1)	Industrial products	5.0g	0.03	1
Acetic anhydride	AR	32ml	0.33	11

Continued

Materials	Specifications	Amount	Mol	Mol ratio
Acetic acid	CP	16ml		
NaHSO$_4$	CP	0.12g	0.001	0.033
Ethanol	CP			

2. Procedures　In a 250ml round bottom flask, guanine(16 – 1)5.0g(0.03mol), NaHSO$_4$ 0.12g(1mmol), acetic anhydride 32ml and acetic acid 16ml were added, and the mixture was heated to reflux at 130℃ for 12h. Then, the refluxing apparatus was changed to a vacuum distillation apparatus and some parts of solvent was removed under vacuum distillation(Notes). The residue was filtered, washed with ethanol and water, and then dried in an oven at 80℃ to obtain a pale yellow powder 4.6g, yield 65.3%.

3. Notes　In this distillation, 2/3 of the solvent in the system should be distilled off, and the residual could be kept for crystallizing fully.

4. Questions

(1) When starting vacuum distillation, why exhaust firstly and then heat and at the end of vacuum distillation, why remove firstly the heat source and then close the pumping?

(2) What is the effect of high refluxing temperature on the reaction system?

Ⅱ. Synthesis of diacetyl acyclovir(DACV)(16 – 3)

1. Materials(Table 16 – 2)

Table 16 – 2　Specification and ratio of raw materials

Materials	Specifications	Amount	Mol	Mol ratio
N,N – diacetylguanine(DAG)(16 – 2)	Prepared in last step	4.6g	0.019	1
(2 – acetoxyethoxy)methyl acetate	CP	7.49g	0.043	2.24
NaHSO$_4$	CP	0.25g	0.002	0.1
Toluene	CP	30ml		

2. Procedures　In a 250ml three – necked flask, N,N – diacetylguanine(DAG)(16 – 2)4.6g (0.019mol), NaHSO$_4$ 0.25g, and toluene 30ml(Note 1) were added and stirred. The mixture was heated to azeotropic reflux and water formed was separated(Note 2). After the completion of the water separation, (2 – acetoxyethoxy)methyl acetate 7.49g(Note 3) was added dropwise, and then the reaction was kept to reflux for 10h. The mixture was then cooled to room temperature. The precipitate was collected by suction filtration, washed with water, and then dried to obtain diacetyl acyclovir(DACV)as a pale yellow powder, 4.3g, yield 71.7%.

3. Notes

Note 1: Both the N atom at the 7 – position and the N atom at the 9 – position in the diacetyl acyclovir(DACV)(16 – 3) could react with(2 – acetoxyethoxy)methyl acetate to produce two different products. When toluene is used as a solvent, the 7 – position substituted by – products reduced.

Note 2: With the water separator, the toluene vapor and water vapor in the azeotropic reflux mixture were condensed and then enter the water separator to remove the water formed in the reaction. The toluene vapor in azeotropic reflux mixture was condensed in the the upper layer of the water separator and would return into the flask.

Note 3: This reaction apparatus is a closed system, and a constant pressure dropping funnel is used to prevent evaporation of the solvent vapor.

4. Questions

(1) How to use the water separator, what should be payed more attention in its operation?

(2) Please give an explanation for the mechanism of this step synthesis.

Ⅲ. Synthesis of acyclovir

1. Materials(Table 16 – 3)

Table 16 – 3   Specification and ratio of raw materials

Materials	Specifications	Amount	Mol	Mol ratio
Diacetyl acyclovir(DACV)(16 – 3)	Prepared in last step	4.3g	0.014	1
Na_2CO_3	AR	1.4g	0.13	10
Water		30ml		
18mol/L hydrochloric acid	Self – prepared			

2. Procedures   In a 250ml three – necked flask, diacetyl acyclovir(DACV)(16 – 3)4.3g, Na_2CO_3 1.4g and H_2O 30ml were added. The mixture was then heated to reflux for 2h and then filtered while hot(Note 1). The filtrate was adjusted to pH 7 using 18mol/L hydrochloric acid(Note 2). A large amount of white solid was appeared, collected by filtration, washed using water and dried. A white powder was obtained 2.11g, yield 69.2%.

3. Notes

Note 1: The solubility of the product changes with temperature, the temperature increases, and the its solubility increases. The product is retained in the filtrate while hot filtration to achieve separation from impurities.

Note 2: When the filtrate solution was adjusted with hydrochloric acid to form sodium salt, the handling of reaction become more simple. It is possible to avoid the loss of the product by slowly adding acid to adjust filtration pH.

4. Questions　According to this reaction, what could be hydrolyzed in diacetyl acyclovir (DACV) (16 – 3)? Give an explanation.

【Characterization of Acyclovir】

Melting point:255.5 ~ 257℃.

^{1}H – NMR:Conformed(Attached figure 16 – 1).

HRMS(ESI $^+$):226.11(M + H $^+$)(Attached figure 16 – 2).

HPLC purity:99.9%

HPLC conditions:

Column:C18(4.6mm × 250mm,5μm).

Detection wavelength:254nm.

Column temperature:35℃.

Mobile phase A: water. Mobile phase B: methanol, and gradient washing was performed according to the Table 16 – 4.

Table 16 – 4　Elution gradient

Time/min	Mobile phase A/%	Mobile phase B/%
0	94	6
15	94	6
40	65	35
41	94	6
51	94	6

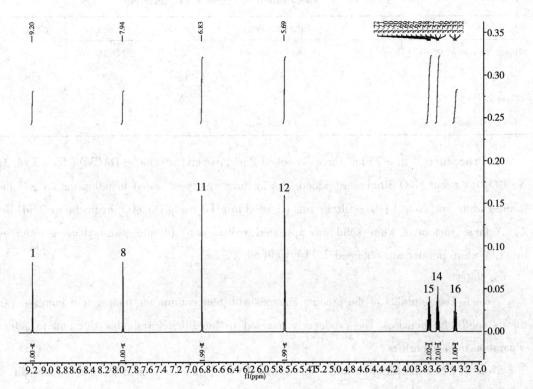

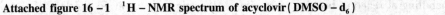

Attached figure 16 – 1　^{1}H – NMR spectrum of acyclovir(DMSO – d$_6$)

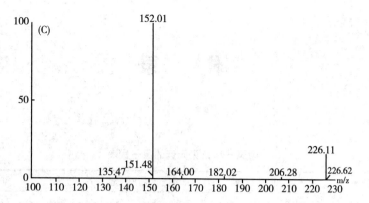

Attached figure 16 – 2　HRMS spectrum of acyclovir(ESI⁺)

附　录

附录一　常见元素的原子量表

元素	符号	原子量	元素	符号	原子量	元素	符号	原子量
铝	Al	26.9815	锗	Ge	72.59	钾	K	39.102
锑	Sb	121.75	金	Au	196.9665	硒	Se	78.96
砷	As	74.9216	氢	H	1.008	硅	Si	28.086
钡	Ba	137.34	碘	I	126.9045	银	Ag	107.868
铍	Be	9.0122	铁	Fe	55.847	钠	Na	22.9898
铋	Bi	208.9806	铅	Pb	207.20	锶	Sr	87.62
溴	Br	79.904	锂	Li	6.941	硫	S	32.06
硼	B	10.81	镁	Mg	24.305	碲	Te	127.60
镉	Cd	112.40	锰	Mn	54.938	钍	Th	232.0381
钙	Ca	40.08	汞	Hg	200.59	锡	Sn	118.69
碳	C	12.011	钼	Mo	95.94	钛	Ti	47.90
铈	Ce	140.12	镍	Ni	58.71	钨	W	183.85
氯	Cl	35.453	氮	N	14.0067	铀	U	238.029
铬	Cr	51.996	氧	O	15.9994	钒	V	50.9414
钴	Co	58.9332	钯	Pd	106.4	锌	Zn	65.37
铜	Cu	63.546	磷	P	30.9738	锆	Zr	91.22
氟	F	18.9984	铂	Pt	195.09			

附录二　水的蒸气压力和密度（0～35℃）

温度/℃	密度 D_4^t	蒸气压力/mmHg	温度/℃	密度 D_4^t	蒸气压力/mmHg
0	0.99987	4.58	13	0.99940	11.19
1	0.99993	4.92	14	0.99927	11.94
2	0.99997	5.29	15	0.99913	12.73
3	0.99999	5.68	16	0.99997	13.56
4	1.00000	6.09	17	0.99980	14.45
5	0.99999	6.53	18	0.99862	15.38
6	0.99997	7.00	19	0.99843	16.37
7	0.99993	7.49	20	0.99823	17.41
8	0.99988	8.02	21	0.99802	18.50
9	0.99981	8.58	22	0.99780	19.66
10	0.99973	9.18	23	0.99757	29.88
11	0.99963	9.81	24	0.99733	22.18
12	0.99952	10.48	25	0.99708	23.54

续表

温度/℃	密度 D_4^t	蒸气压力/mmHg	温度/℃	密度 D_4^t	蒸气压力/mmHg
26	0.99682	24.99	31	0.99537	33.42
27	9.88655	26.50	32	0.99505	35.37
28	0.99627	28.10	33	0.99473	37.43
29	0.99597	29.78	34	0.99440	39.59
30	0.99568	31.55	35	0.99406	41.85

附录三 常用的冰盐浴冷却剂

盐	每100g碎冰用盐/g	冷却剂温度降低到/℃
$NaNO_3$	50	−18.5
NaCl	33	−21.2
NaCl NH_4Cl } 混合物	40 20 }	−26
NH_4Cl $NaNO_3$ } 混合物	13 37.5 }	−30.7
K_2CO_3	33	−46
$CaCl_2 \cdot 6H_2O$	143	−35

配制冷却剂可用碎冰或雪，盐要预先冷到0℃。

附录四 其他冷却剂和最低冷却温度

冷却剂	最低冷却温度/℃	冷却剂	最低冷却温度/℃
冰	0	三氯甲烷/N_2	−63
乙二醇/CO_2	−15	三氯甲烷/CO_2	−63
冰（100）/NH_4Cl（25）	−15	乙醇/CO_2	−72
冰（100）/NaCl（33）	−21	乙醚/CO_2	−77
四氯化碳/N_2	−23	丙酮/CO_2	−78
四氯化碳/CO_2	−23	甲醇/N_2	−98
冰（100）/EtOH（100）	−30	n-戊烷/N_2	−131
乙腈/N_2	−41	N_2	−180
冰（100）/$CaCl_2$（150）	−49		

附录五 常用的盐浴

盐	溶于100g水中的量/g	溶液的沸点/℃
NaCl	40.7	108 ~ 109
NH_4Cl	87.1	114.8 ~ 115
K_2CO_3	202.5	133.5
$CaCl_2$	305	178

附录六 常用干燥剂的分类及使用方法

分类	干燥剂	适用的物质和条件	不适用的物质条件	干燥原理	特点	使用方法	备注
金属、金属氢化物	Mg	醇类				无水 MeOH 的制备：MeOH 和 Mg 一起加热回流，然后蒸馏出 MeOH	不要蒸馏到干
	Na	烷烃、芳烃、醚类	用于卤代烃时，有爆炸的危险，不适用于醇、酯、酸、醛、酮、胺类的干燥	$\rightarrow NaOH + H_2$	干燥能力高，但在表面易覆盖 NaOH 致效果下降，脱水能力小	切成薄片或压成丝状，放入待干燥液体中。对 THF 和 Et_2O 也可加入 Pb_2CO 和 Na 回流再进行蒸馏	和水反应生成 H_2，与大量水接触会燃烧，保存和处理时要注意。蒸馏时要蒸干。用过的 Na 用乙醇分解破坏
	CaH_2	烃类、卤代烃、t-丁醇、三级胺、THF、DMSO、吡啶等	醛、酮、羧酸	$\rightarrow Ca(OH)_2 + H_2$	脱水容量大、处理方便、适用范围广	加入 CaH_2，在 Ar 或 N_2 气流中蒸馏，或者将粒状的 CaH_2 加到液体中进行干燥	和水反应产生 H_2，保存和处理上要注意
	$LiAlH_4$	醚类、乙醚、THF 等	易和酸、胺、硫醇、乙炔等含活波氢的化合物及酮、酯、酰氯、酰胺、腈、硝基化合物、环氧氯、烯丙醇等高沸点化合物	$\rightarrow LiOH + Al(OH)_3 + H_2$	同时能分解待干燥物中的醇、羰基化合物、过氧化物	加入 $LiAlH_4$，在 Ar 或 N_2 气流中蒸馏	$LiAlH_4$ 在 125℃ 时分解，蒸馏时不要蒸干，过量的 $LiAlH_4$ 用氯化铵溶液或乙酸乙酯分解。保存时不要与水和 CO_2 接触
中性干燥剂	Na_2SO_4 $MgSO_4$ $CaSO_4$	几乎全部溶剂	Na_2SO_4 在 33℃ 以上，$MgSO_4$ 在 48℃ 以上释放出结晶水，因此不适合在以上温度使用	$\rightarrow Na_2SO_4 \cdot 10H_2O$ $\rightarrow MgSO_4 \cdot 7H_2O$ $\rightarrow CaSO_4 \cdot \frac{1}{2}H_2O$	Na_2SO_4 脱水容量大、速度慢，$MgSO_4$ 脱水容量大、脱水速度比 Na_2SO_4 快，$CaSO_4$ 脱水容量小，但脱水力强、速度快	加到待干燥液体中	$CaSO_4$ 在 235℃ 加热 2~3 小时后可以再生
	$CuSO_4$	乙醇、苯、乙醚等	能和甲醇反应，所以不能用于甲醇干燥	$\rightarrow CuSO_4 \cdot 5H_2O$	无水物呈白色，与结晶水合物呈蓝色	加到待干燥液体中	
	$CaCl_2$	烃类、卤代烃、醚类、中性气体等	醇、胺、酰胺酮、氨基酸、酯、酸等	$\rightarrow CaCl_2 \cdot 6H_2O$	吸水速度慢，30℃ 以下生成六水合物，脱水容量大，有潮解性	加入到待干燥液体中，加入干燥器，干燥管中使用	

146

分类	干燥剂	适用的物质和条件	不适用的物质条件	干燥原理	特点	使用方法	备注
中性干燥剂	活化氧化铝	烃、醚类、三氯甲烷、苯、吡啶等		吸附	同时能除去醚类中的过氧化物，处理方便，吸收力大	做成填充柱，让溶剂通过	175℃以上加热6～8小时可以再生。加热到800℃以上变成活性氧化铝
	硅胶（蓝色）	几乎全部固体和气体物质		$\rightarrow SiO_2 \cdot xH_2O$	处理方便，脱水力极强，无水时蓝色，吸水后粉红色	加入干燥器，干燥管中使用	150℃以上加热2～3小时可以再生
	分子筛	卤代烃、醚类、THF、二噁烷、丙酮、吡啶、DMF、DMSO、HMPA等，适用范围 pH 5～11	对强酸、碱性物质不稳定	结晶空隙吸水	随干燥时间长而脱水力显著高，高温时，吸附力也不降低	加入到待干燥溶剂瓶中，根据结晶的孔径不同，溶剂进行选择使用	350℃加热3小时再生
碱性干燥剂	KOH NaOH	胺类等碱性物质，中性或碱性气体	酸、醛、酮、醇、酯等		脱水速度快，脱水力大。易潮解	加到液体、干燥皿、干燥管中	
	Na_2CO_3 K_2CO_3	胺类等碱性物质，醇、酮酯、腈等	酸	$\rightarrow K_2CO_3 \cdot 2H_2O$		加到液体中，适合预干燥	可加热熔化、活化
	CaO	胺类等碱性物质，醇等	酸	$\rightarrow Ca(OH)_2$	脱水速度小，便宜，可大量使用，能吸收 CO_2	加到液体，干燥皿、干燥管中。块状可粉碎使用	细的粉末物中，$Ca(OH)_2$、$CaCO_3$ 为主、干燥能力低
酸性干燥剂	H_2SO_4	Br_2 中性气体	醇、酚、酮、乙烯等		吸收速度、容量大、吸水后浓度降低后、干燥能力急剧下降	加到干燥皿、气体干燥瓶中	
	P_2O_5	烃、卤烃、酸酐、腈、中性气体	碱性物质、酮、醇、胺、酰胺、卤化氢、丙酮	$\rightarrow$偏磷酸等	吸水速度、吸水能力最大。在表面上形成偏磷酸膜时，效率变低、白色粉末、难处理	加到干燥皿、干燥管中、多用于固体、气体干燥	P_2O_5 的后处理、用乙醇分解或自然放置让其吸湿潮解

147

附录七 常用溶剂的物理常数

溶剂	沸点/℃ (760mmHg)	熔点/℃	分子量	密度 (20℃)	介电常数	溶解度 /(g/100g 水①)	和水的共沸混合物		闪点/℃	阈限值 (×10⁻⁶)
							bp./℃	% H₂O		
乙醚	35	-116	74	0.71	4.3	6.0	34	1	-45	400
戊烷	36	-130	72	0.63	1.8	不溶	35	1	-40	500
二氯甲烷	40	-95	85	1.33	8.9	1.30	39	2	无	250
二硫化碳	46	-111	86	1.26	2.6	0.29 (20℃)	44	2	-30	20
丙酮	56	-95	58	0.79	20.7	∞	56	—	-18	1000
三氯甲烷	61	-64	119	1.49	4.8	0.82 (20℃)	56	3	无	25
甲醇	65	-98	32	0.79	32.7	∞		—	12	200
四氢呋喃	66	-109	72	0.89	7.6	∞	65	4	-14	200
己烷	69	-95	86	0.66	1.9	不溶	62	6	-26	500
三氟醋酸	72	-15	114	1.49	39.5	∞	105	21	无	—
四氯化碳	77	-23	154	1.59	2.2	0.08	66	4	无	10
醋酸乙酯	77	-84	88	0.9	6.0	8.1	71	8	-4	400
乙醇	78	-114	46	0.79	24.6	∞	78	4	13	1000
环己烷	81	6.5	84	0.78	2.0	0.01	70	8	-17	300
苯	80	5.5	78	0.88	2.3	0.18	69	9	-11	25
甲基乙基酮	80	-87	72	0.8	18.5	24.0 (20℃)	73	11	-1	200
乙腈	82	-44	41	0.78	37.5	∞	77	16	6	40
异丙醇	82	-88	60	0.79	19.9	∞	80	12	12	—
正丁醇	82	26	74	0.78 (30℃)	12.5	∞	80	12	11	100
乙二醇二甲烷	83	-58	90	0.86	7.2	∞	77	10	1	—
三乙胺	90	-115	101	0.73	2.4	10	75	10	-7	25
丙醇	97	-126	60	0.8	20.3	∞	88	28	25	200

续表

溶剂	沸点/℃ (760mmHg)	熔点/℃	分子量	密度 (20℃)	介电常数	溶解度 /(g/100g水①)	和水的共沸混合物 bp./℃	和水的共沸混合物 % H₂O	闪点/℃	阈限值 (×10⁻⁶)
甲基环己烷	101	-127	98	0.77	2.0	0.01	80	24.1	-6	500
甲酸	101	8	46	1.22	58.5	∞	107	26	—	5
硝基甲烷	101	-29	61	1.14	35.9	11.1	84	24	-41	100
1,4-二氧己环	101	12	88	1.03	2.2	∞	88	18	12	50
甲苯	111	-95	92	0.87	2.4	0.05	85	20	4	100
吡啶	115	-42	79	0.98	12.4	∞	94	42	23	5
正丁醇	118	-89	74	0.81	17.5	7.45	93	43	29	100
醋酸	118	17	60	1.05	6.2	∞	无	—	40	10
乙二醇单甲醚	125	-85	76	0.96	16.9	∞	100	85	42	25
吗啉	129	-3	87	1.00	7.4	∞	无	—	38	20
氯苯	132	-46	113	1.11	5.6	0.05 (30℃)	90	28	29	75
醋酐	140	-73	102	1.08	20.7	反应	—	—	53	5
二甲苯（混合体）	138~142	13②	106	0.86	2③	0.02	93	33	38	—
二丁醚	142	-95	130	0.77	3.1	0.03 (20℃)	93	33	38	—
均四氯乙烷	146	-44	168	1.59	8.2	0.29 (20℃)	94	34	无	5
二苯甲醚	154	-38	108	0.99	4.3	1.04	96	41	—	—
二甲基甲酰胺	153	-60	73	0.95	36.7	∞	无	—	67	10
二甘醇二甲醚	160	—	134	0.94	—	∞	100	78	63	—
1,3,5-三甲基苯	165	-45	120	0.87	2.3	0.03 (20℃)	97	—	95	—
二甲亚砜	189	18	78	1.1	46.7	25.3	无	—	95	—
二甘醇单甲醚	194	-76	120	1.02	—	∞	无	—	93	—
乙二醇	197	-16④ -13	62	1.11	37.7	∞	无	—	116	100

续表

| 溶剂 | 沸点/℃ (760mmHg) | 熔点/℃ | 分子量 | 密度 (20℃) | 介电常数 | 溶解度 /(g/100g水①) | 和水的共沸混合物 | | 闪点/℃ | 阈限值 (×10⁻⁶) |
							bp./℃	% H₂O		
N-甲基-2-吡咯烷酮	202	-24	99	1.03	32	∞	—	—	96	—
硝基苯	211	6	123	1.2	34.8	0.19 (20℃)	99	88	88	1
甲酰胺	210	3	45	1.13	111	∞	—	—	154	20
六甲基磷酰三胺	233	7	179	1.03	30	∞	—	—	—	—
喹啉	237	-15	129	1.09	9	0.6 (20℃)	—	97	—	—
二甘醇	245	-7	106	1.11	31.7	∞	—	—	—	—
二苯醚	258	27	170	1.07	3.7 (>27℃)	0.39	100	96	205	—
三甘醇	288	-4	150	1.12	23.7	∞	无	—	166	—
丁砜	287	28	120	1.26 (30℃)	43	∞ (30℃)	无	—	177	—
甘油	290	18	92	1.26	42.5	∞	无	—	177	—
三乙醇胺	335	22	149	1.12 (25℃)	29.4	∞	—	—	179	—
邻苯二甲酸二丁酯	340	-35	278	1.05	6.4	不溶	无	—	171	5

注：①除非另作注明，皆为25℃的溶解度。溶解度<0.01作为不溶解。
②对二甲苯的熔点（较高熔点的异构体）。
③近似值。
④因为很容易过冷和形成玻璃状，所以有两种熔点。

附录八　常用溶剂的提纯、干燥和贮藏

溶剂	沸点/℃ （容许沸距）	初步提纯	进一步的干燥和提纯	贮藏
戊烷 己烷 环己烷 其他烷烃	36 (2~3) 69 (2.5)① 80.7 (1)	必要时，首先用浓硫酸洗涤几次，以除去烯烃；然后水洗，用 $CaCl_2$ 干燥，蒸馏，收集潮湿的前馏分之后的正沸物	几乎没有进一步处理的必要；一定要处理时，可利用恒沸蒸馏脱水	500ml 以内贮藏于带塞的试剂瓶中；大量和长期贮藏时应采用螺旋盖的棕色瓶，向其中加入分子筛是没有意义的
苯② 甲苯② 邻二甲苯 间二甲苯 对二甲苯	80.1 (0.5) 110.6 (1) 144.5 139 138.3 (1)	$CaCl_2$ 干燥，分馏、弃去前面 5%~10% 的潮湿的前馏分	重蒸，分去前面 5% 的馏分	500ml 以内贮藏于带塞的试剂瓶中；大量和长期贮藏时应采用螺旋盖的棕色瓶，向其中加入分子筛是没有意义的
二氯甲烷 三氯甲烷 四氯化碳 1，2-二氯乙烷	40 (1) 61.2 (0.5) 76.8 (0.5) 83.5 (1)	水洗，$CaCl_2$ 干燥，蒸馏，弃去前面 5% 的潮湿的前馏分	加入 P_2O_5 重蒸：在小量和特殊的情况下可通过氧化铝（碱性，一级活性）直接放入反应瓶	500ml 以内贮藏于带塞的试剂瓶中；大量和长期贮藏时应采用螺旋盖的棕色瓶，向其中加入分子筛是没有意义的。长期贮藏的三氯甲烷，应放在密闭的瓶中，装满，并保存于黑暗处
乙醚 二异丙基醚	34.5 (1) 68.5 (1)	检查是否含有过氧化物。如证实其存在，用 5% 偏亚硫酸氢钠溶液洗涤，然后以饱和 NaCl 溶液洗涤，用 $CaCl_2$ 干燥，蒸馏（不能用浓硫酸）	小量：通过相当于其重量 10% 的氧化铝（碱性，一级活性）蒸入反应瓶	装于有螺旋盖的金属容器中，几乎装满，置于阴凉黑暗处，长期贮藏时应加以密封③
四氢呋喃 1，2-二甲氧基乙烷（甘醇）	65.5 (0.5) 84 (1)④	加入 KOH，放置过夜，倾泻，做过氧化物试验。如呈阳性，则加入最多 0.4% 重量的 $NaBH_4$ 搅拌过夜。加入 CaH_2 蒸馏，但不能蒸干	在氩气保护下加入金属钾蒸馏；少量的可通过氧化铝（碱性，一级活性）直接放入反应瓶	盛于干燥的塑料瓶中，加入碱性的活性氧化铝，并用氩气保护；长期贮藏时，必须加以密封
二噁烷	101.5 (1)④ (mp.11~12)	加入 KOH，放置过夜，倾泻，做过氧化物试验。如呈阳性，则加入最多 0.4% 重量的 $NaBH_4$ 搅拌过夜。加入 CaH_2 蒸馏，但不能蒸干	加入金属钠，在氩气保护下蒸馏	盛于干燥的塑料瓶中，加入碱性的活性氧化铝，并用氩气保护；长期贮藏时，必须加以密封，最好冷冻，保存于冰箱中
二硫化碳	46.5 (1)	加入少量 P_2O_5，蒸馏，使用水浴，用蒸汽加热	加入少量汞，振荡，再加入 P_2O_5 重蒸	不要贮藏于实验室内！极易着火
醋酸乙酯 醋酸甲酯	77.1 (0.5) 57 (1)	用活性硫酸钙和（或）无水碳酸钾干燥，倾泻，小心地蒸馏	加入最多 5% 重量的醋酐后分馏	加入 5Å 活性分子筛，密闭保存
其他沸点低于100℃的酯			分馏	
乙腈	81.5 (0.5)④	顺次以 $MgSO_4$ 和无水 K_2CO_3 干燥，倾泻；加入 CaH_2 蒸馏	通过 P_2O_5 分馏；小量：通过氧化铝（碱性，一级活性）直接蒸入反应瓶	加入 3Å 活性分子筛，保存于小瓶中，并标明日期

溶剂	沸点/℃ （容许沸距）	初步提纯	进一步的干燥和提纯	贮藏
丙酮	56.2（0.5）	蒸馏，控制2℃的收集沸程，以无水硫酸钙干燥，倾泻，重蒸	如用于氧化反应，需在回流下加入足够数量的KMnO₄直到紫色不褪为止。蒸馏，干燥，再分馏。通过NaI化合物可以得到很纯的试剂	加入新活化的3Å分子筛 加入新活化的5Å分子筛
2-丁酮	79.5（0.5）	恒沸蒸馏除去水（沸点73.5℃），以无水硫酸钙分别干燥馏出的恒沸物和残余部分，倾泻，重蒸		
甲醇	64.5（0.5）	即使对于工业级产品，简单蒸馏也已足够	经过预干燥后加入CaH₂重蒸，直接蒸入反应瓶	贮藏于小瓶中，加入3Å活性分子筛
乙醇	78.3（0.5）	将95%乙醇与CaO一同回流并蒸馏（CaO的用量至少应达含水量的1.5倍）		
异丙醇	82.5（0.5）	分馏，蒸去恒沸物（沸点80.3℃）之后收集正沸物；对恒沸物的处理与95%乙醇相同		
正丙醇 较高级的醇	97.2（0.5）	分馏，除去含水的恒沸物后，收集正馏分		
叔丁醇	82.5（0.5）（mp.25.8）	水恒沸物的沸点79.9℃，处理与异丙醇相同	与前述的醇相同，但蒸馏时，需防止产物凝结于冷凝管中导致堵塞	与前述的醇相同，但冷天最好保存于温暖处，以免固化
乙二醇 较高级的二醇	198,68~70/533.2Pa 108~110/3732.4Pa（2）	真空分馏，弃去5%~10%的前馏分。注意，其蒸发潜热很大	溶入1%重量的金属钠，重新分馏	分装于小塑料瓶中，但冷天保存于温暖处，以免固化
硝基甲烷 硝基乙烷	101.3（1）[3]115	CaCl₂干燥，倾泻，分馏	加入4Å分子筛，重蒸	加入4Å分子筛贮藏
甲酸	101（1）（mp.8.3）	分馏，最好稍作减压。加入邻苯二甲酸酐，回流后重蒸能获得进一步干燥。与水恒沸物的沸点107℃，含水22.5%	将经过纯化的试剂完全冷冻，再让其温热，熔化总量的10%~20%，倾出液化部分，使用剩下的试剂。全部操作应在脱水的条件下完成	贮藏于有螺旋盖的瓶中
乙酸	118（0.5）（mp.16.6）	加入总量5%的醋酐和2%的CrO₃后分馏		
吡啶甲基吡啶	115.5（0.5）	向粗品中加入KOH，倾泻，分馏	加入CaO、BaO或活性很强的碱性氧化铝，重新分馏	加入5Å分子筛密闭保存，并注明日期

溶剂	沸点/℃（容许沸距）	初步提纯	进一步的干燥和提纯	贮藏
N，N – 二甲基甲酰胺⑥	153，42/1333Pa 55/2666Pa（1）	真空分馏，弃去前面和最后各10%的馏分；避免常压蒸馏	加入 CaO、BaO 或氧化铝（碱性，一级活性）搅拌过夜，再次真空分馏	加入新活化的分子筛，贮藏于小瓶中，并注明日期。大量贮藏超过 500ml 时，考虑到多次开启将有水汽渗入，应加入大量的分子筛
N，N – 二甲基乙酰胺	166，58～59/1466.3Pa 63/2399.4Pa（1）			
N，N – 甲基吡咯烷酮	202，78～79/1333Pa 96～97/3199.2Pa（1）			
二甲基亚砜	190，50/340Pa 72/1360Pa 84～85/2932.6Pa（1）（mp.8.5）		加入 CaH_2 搅拌过夜，然后从中减压分馏；如已足够干燥，可通过部分冷冻而进一步提纯	
六甲基磷酰三胺	235，68～70/133.3Pa 115/1200Pa 126/3999Pa（1）（mp.7）		加入 CaH_2，于 100℃下减压搅拌 1 小时，然后真空分馏	分装于小的（50ml）塑料瓶中，加入活化的13Å分子筛或除去了矿物油的 NaH，并以氩气保护

注：①低质的廉价己烷。

②假定其中没有含硫化合物，如噻吩等。

③加入相当于总量0.001%的二羟基酚，可使其稳定化；即使已产生少量过氧化物，亦能使其重新稳定。

④市售品的纯度常常不合要求，纯化需特别仔细。

⑤溶剂中可能有部分与水形成的低沸恒沸物。

⑥据报道，该试剂对光敏感，最好始终贮藏于棕色瓶中。